A colour atlas of

General Surgical

Diagnosis

WILLIAM F. WALKER

DSc, ChM, FRCS, FRCS (Ed), FRSE

Consultant Surgeon
Ninewells Hospital, Dundee
Honorary Reader in Surgery
Dundee University

WOLFE MEDICAL PUBLICATIONS LTD

Copyright © William F. Walker, 1976
Published by Wolfe Medical Publications Ltd., 1976
Printed by Smeets-Weert, Holland,
ISBN 0 7234 0404 6
4th impression 1984

General Editor, Wolfe Medical Books
G. Barry Carruthers MD (Lond)

This book is one of the titles in the series of
Wolfe Medical Atlases, a series which brings together
probably the world's largest systematic published
collection of diagnostic colour photographs.
  For a full list of Atlases in the series, plus
forthcoming titles and details of our surgical, dental
and veterinary Atlases, please write to
Wolfe Medical Publications Ltd, Wolfe House,
3 Conway Street, London W1P 6HE.

Acknowledgements

I wish to acknowledge my indebtedness to many of my colleagues in Dundee for the use of their photographs. These include my colleagues in the Departments of Surgery, Medicine, Radiology, Dermatology, Radiotherapy, Dentistry, Plastic Surgery, Forensic Medicine and Pathology. The quality of the pathological photographs reflects the skill of Mr R Fox. The clinical and radiological photographs were kindly done by Mr M Ettle and Mr T King.

I am also indebted to friends outside Dundee for their help; Professor A P M Forrest, Mr T McNair and Mr James Thompson in Edinburgh, Professor I D A Johnson in Newcastle, and Mr J Gazet and Dr A Wisdom in London.

The line drawings were done by Miss M Benstead, the medical artist.

To Bettie, Bill, Chris and Fiona

Table of Contents

Introduction

This atlas is based on a series of meetings held in the last term of medical students' final year. The object of these meetings was to review many conditions which might appear in their final examinations. A slide (clinical, radiological or pathological) of a condition was projected onto a screen and this acted as a 'hat-peg' on which to base discussion on aetiology, pathology, diagnosis and treatment. As many illustrations were shown, the discussions revolved mainly around diagnosis and treatment.

The material presented has been enlarged to cover most of the conditions seen in general surgery. Although designed primarily for final year medical students, it should prove of benefit throughout the clinical part of the medical and dental undergraduate training and even as a refresher course for those sitting the higher surgical examinations. General practitioners may also find some help in unusual cases presenting in their surgery, and nurses, who have much of the care of these patients, should find it of interest.

An atlas is a pictorial representation and not a general textbook of surgery. It should be regarded as an accompaniment to the written word, as surgical diagnosis should not be based on a spot diagnosis however attractive it is as a short cut. It must be based on the taking of a complete history and careful clinical examination supplemented by various investigations.

In assembling the collection of illustrations I am indebted to the generosity of many individuals not mentioned individually in the acknowledgements. Even with their help it has not been possible to cover rare conditions thoroughly, although a few are included on the basis that they were available.

Non-specific Infections

The diagnosis of infection of skin and subcutaneous tissues is largely dependent on recognition by sight with some reliance on history, occupation, and specific investigations. Infection is mainly of bacterial origin, but other causes include virus agents, yeasts, fungi, protozoa and infestation by insects.

1 Boil (furuncle, folliculitis) This is an infection of a hair follicle by the staphylococcus. The infection spreads to the tissue around the follicle and proceeds to suppuration. Common sites are the back of the finger or neck, the eyelash, the nose, external auditory meatus and peri-anal area.

2 A boil in the nostril is very dangerous as infection may spread by the angular vein to the ophthalmic plexus and thence to the cavernous sinus producing a cavernous sinus thrombosis.

3 Cavernous sinus thrombosis in this patient followed a septic blister on the upper lip. The diagnosis is based on a primary infection in the dangerous area – upper lip and nose – followed by an acute onset of pyrexia, toxicity, going on to delirium and coma. Gross oedema of the conjunctiva and eyelids occurs with swelling of the side of the face. A progressive exophthalmos develops with ophthalmoplegia. The condition may spread to the other side.

4 Sycosis barbae is due to the spread of the staphylococci from follicle to follicle. The examples seen today are usually of a mild form as shown here.

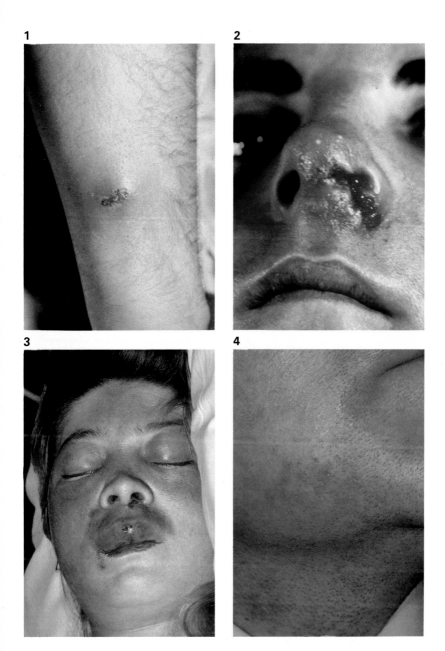

5 Carbuncle This lesion is now fortunately less common. In this example the staphylococcal infection has involved a number of hair follicles and has spread into the subcutaneous tissue.

6 Skin necrosis with a black area develops if the carbuncle is not properly treated. The skin eventually sloughs off leaving a large ulcer. It is, or was, especially common in poorly controlled diabetes.

7 An abscess is defined as a localised collection of pus. In the peripheral tissues it is often due to the staphylococcus but in the abdominal area may be due to *E. Coli*. The superficial abscess shown here has all the characteristics of inflammation: pain, redness, swelling, tenderness. An extra sign of the abscess is fluctuation elicited by pressing the fingers in two places on the swelling and again at right angles to previous points. Where thick fascia covers the abscess, as here in the neck, fluctuation may be a late sign.

8 A superficial abscess may denote deep seated infection as in this case where the abscess was noted in the upper thigh and when opened a tract led down to the upper end of femur.

5

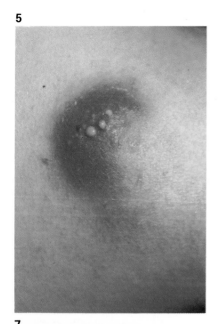

6

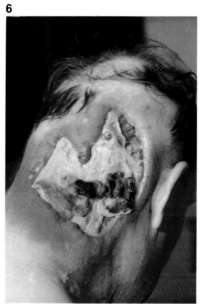

7

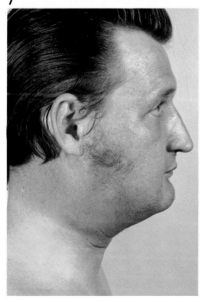

8

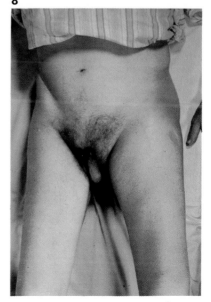

9 A cellulitis is a spreading inflammation in the cellular tissue plane due to infection by the streptococcus. The leg is a common site. Apart from the usual signs of inflammation the diagnostic points are that the skin is not sharply raised and the redness extends in the tissues with no well demarcated edge. In this it resembles a 'blush' – albeit a painful one!

10 Orbital cellulitis may spread from the maxilla into the soft tissues of the orbit. Thus the maxilla should be x-rayed. There is danger of spread of the infection to the eye, meninges, or cavernous sinus.

11 'Ludwig's' angina is a cellulitis under the deep cervical fascia of the neck. The gross swelling can elevate the tongue and cause oral obstruction. Anaesthesia in such a patient can be difficult and dangerous.

12 Erysipelas is sometimes confused with cellulitis. It is a streptococcal infection of the skin and subcutaneous tissues and is characterised by an obvious raised edge to the red area. This edge can often be felt more easily than seen.

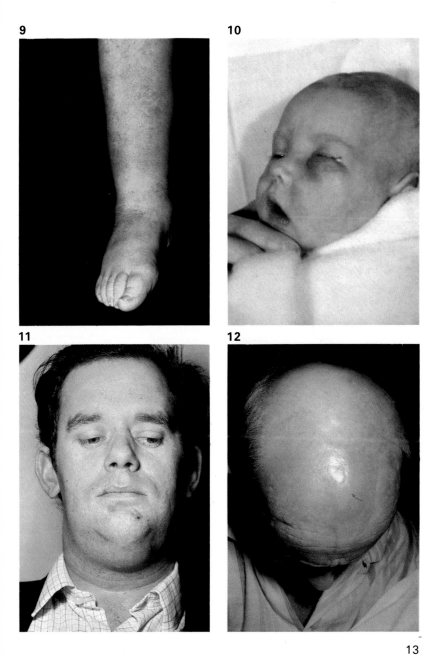

9

10

11

12

13 Pulp infection is one of the commonest types of hand infection, here shown affecting the distal part of the thumb. Necrosis of the skin is beginning. Spread to the tendon sheath would be serious.

14 A pulp granuloma may occur where infection has not been eliminated completely. Exuberant granulation tissue is evident.

15 Anthrax This lesion occurred on the neck of a farm worker who carried sacks of bone meal on his shoulder. It started as an itchy swelling which increased in size. The centre broke down leaving a characteristic black slough with a ring of small vesicles round it. Lymph nodes were involved. Anthrax bacillus was isolated from a smear of the fluid of a vesicle.

16 Anthrax adentis The gross swelling of the face and glands is apparent with toxaemia. Temperature and pulse were elevated. This patient also had contact with bone meal. Other types of anthrax infection are the pulmonary form (wool sorter's disease) and a less common alimentary form which resembles cholera.

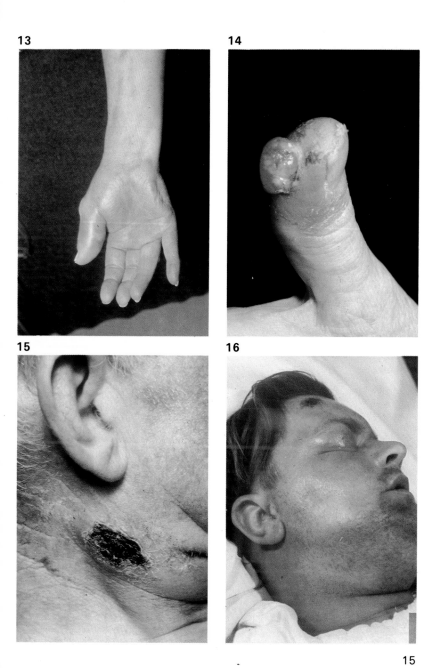

13

14

15

16

17 Actinomycosis is not a common condition but is seen most often in the head and neck, less so in the thorax and the abdomen. It begins as a hard, slowly enlarging nodule which may break down with multiple sinuses. The 'sulphur granules' in the pus are diagnostic. Biopsy may be necessary and shows the typical picture.

18 Actinomycosis of upper pulp in the jaw Biopsy shows the two central masses of Ray fungus.

19 Actinomycosis of the lower jaw There is slight redness of the skin, and a tumour mass infiltrating the tissues. A healed sinus is seen near the centre.

20 Risus sardonicus due to tetanus This child presented with general malaise, pyrexia and a rapid pulse. Next day muscular spasms occurred. The entry wound was slight.

21 A small puncture wound occurred 10 days before the onset of the tetanus seen in the patient in **20**.

17

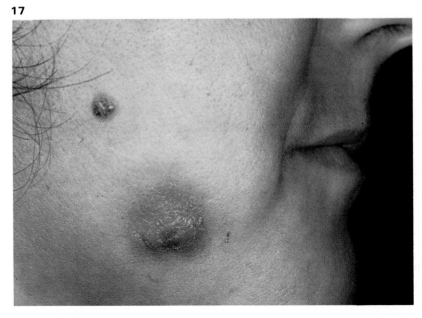

18

19

20

21

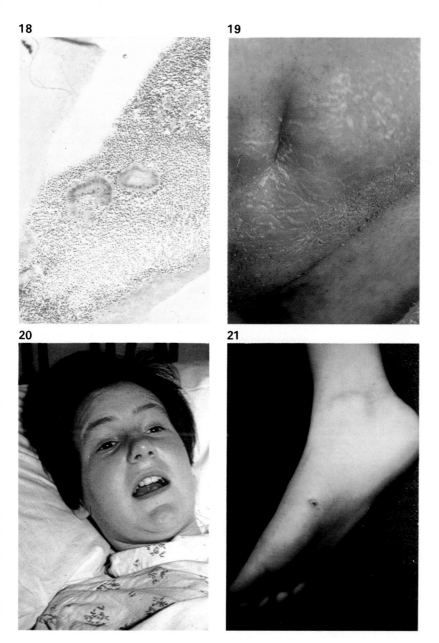

22 The shingles lesion due to *herpes zoster* is sometimes seen in the surgical patient who appears to have an 'acute abdomen'. The vesicular, painful tender eruption along the course of a nerve is diagnostic.

22

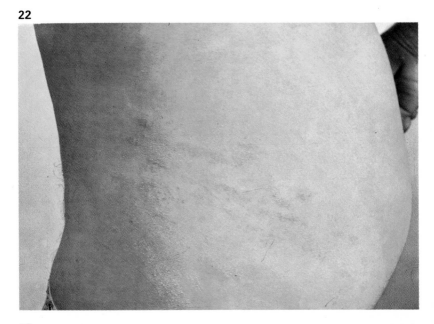

Tumours of the Skin

Benign
Papilloma
Condyloma
Molluscum contagiosum
Haemangioma, capillary
Haemangioma, cavernous
Melanotic naevus
Sebaceous cyst
Implantation cyst
Keratoacanthoma
Keloid
Cutaneous horn

Malignant
Squamous epithelioma
Basal cell carcinoma
Malignant melanoma
Kaposi's sarcoma
Metastases

Premalignant
Bowen's disease
Lentigo
Lentigo maligna
Solar keratosis
Arsenical keratosis
Leucoplakia
Radiodermatitis
Erythema ab igne
Marjolin's ulcer
Varicose ulcer
Sebaceous cyst
Lupus vulgaris

Skin changes in malignancy
Acanthosis nigricans
Pemphigoid
Pigmentation of lips
Dermatomyositis
Erythroderma
Carcinoid facies
Herpes zoster

Benign tumours

23 Papilloma or wart is composed typically of a central axis of connective tissue, blood vessels and lymphatics covered by squamous epithelium. It is raised entirely above the surface and the base is circumscribed.

24 Papilloma of face This illustrates that the lesion may extend over a large area. The branching processes are distinct here but may be closely blended together in smaller ones.

25 Condyloma The lesion is usually multiple, sessile, and has a moist excoriated surface which discharges a watery secretion. It is found at the corner of the mouth and more commonly around the anus and vulva. It is usually of viral origin, but the fluid from the surface should be examined for spirochaetes.

26 Molluscum contagiosum These are small nodules raised above the surface, occurring in clusters. They are umbilicated and have a pearly or waxy appearance and as shown here are common in children. The contents of a papule should be examined for 'molluscum bodies'.

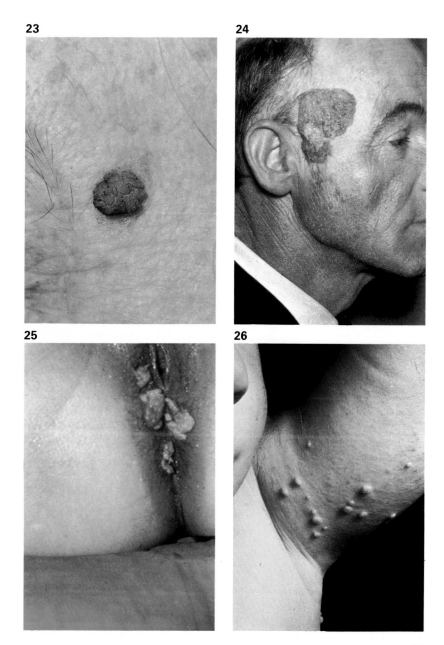

27 Haemangioma, capillary The 'port-wine' stain is flat and varies in colour from pink to bright red. It is present at birth and does not regress with age. It may be associated with similar lesions in the nervous system.

28 Haemangioma, cavernous (strawberry naevus) appears shortly after birth and grows slowly for months. On compression it empties and refills on release of pressure. Spontaneous regression usually occurs by the age of 10 years.

29 Haemangioma, cavernous This lesion may occur in the subcutaneous tissue and infiltrate the surrounding tissues. Ulceration and bleeding may occur and can be serious.

30 Melanotic naevus (pigmented mole) This lesion appears particularly on the face and trunk especially around puberty. The size and degree of pigmentation varies. It tends to grow slowly. Rapid growth, increased pigmentation, ulceration or bleeding may indicate change to a malignant melanoma. Complete excision biopsy is then required.

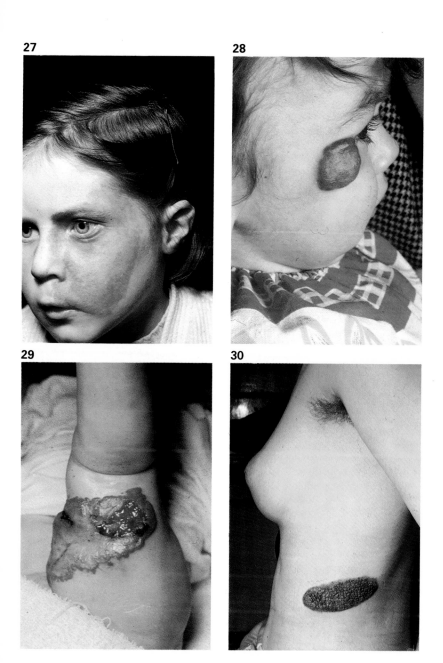

27

28

29

30

31 Sebaceous cyst This may be single or multiple and is common in the scalp of adults. The swelling is rounded, firm when small and softer when large and may even be fluctuant. It is adherent to the skin and freely mobile over bone. Infection of these cysts is common.

32 Implantation cyst is seen in barbers as in this case, or in seamstresses. It is painless cystic swelling which appears slowly on the palmar surface of the fingers. The punctum of entry is seen in the middle of the cyst.

33 Keratoacanthoma (molluscum sebaceum) is a rapidly growing tumour formed usually on the face or other light exposed areas. From papule to large size as shown here may take only two months. The symmetrical shape and crateriform plug of keratin are characteristic.

34 Keratoacanthoma of nose might easily be mistaken for a carcinoma. The rapid growth and volcanic-like appearance serve to distinguish it.

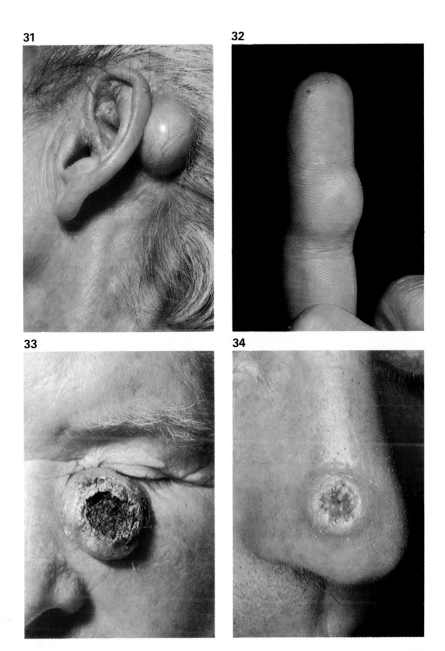

31

32

33

34

35 Keloid This overgrowth of connective tissue in a scar is particularly common in Africans but in Europe may be seen in burns as here.

36 Cutaneous horn This is an excessive form of keratosis where hard accretions of keratin build up to form a horn.

37 A ganglion arises from synovial membrane or capsule of a joint. It is commonly seen near the wrist. The site and the smooth firm semi-cystic feel suggest the diagnosis.

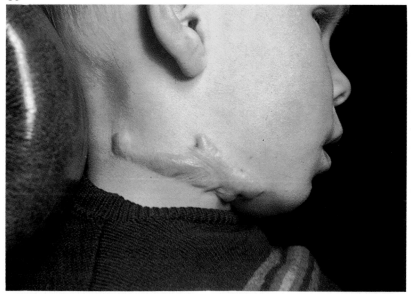

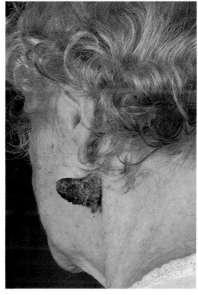

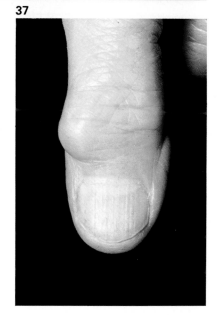

Malignant tumours

38 Squamous epithelioma of hand begins as a nodule and at that stage is difficult to diagnose. Diagnosis is easier when it is fixed to and infiltrates the skin and deeper tissues and ulceration occurs. The ulcer has thick edges, an irregular granular base, and a serous discharge. Lymphatic glands may be enlarged.

39 Squamous epithelioma of ear This is a common site. The lesion has the typical characteristics.

40 Basal cell carcinoma (rodent ulcer) This begins as a nodular area with one or more pearly nodules enlarging slowly.

41 A further extension of the same lesion still without ulceration.

38

39

40

41

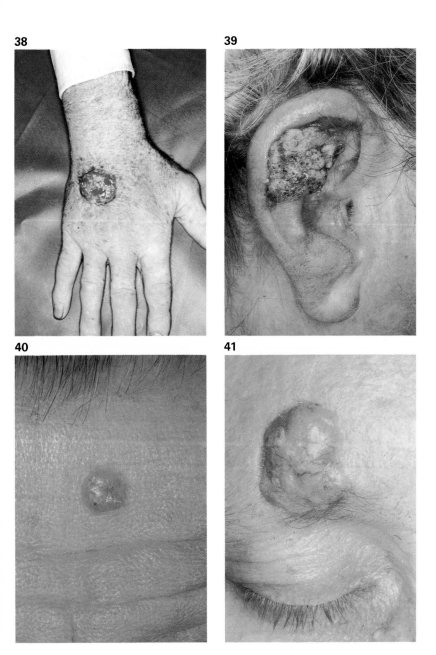

42 Basal cell carcinoma of the forehead shows a shallow ulcer with very narrow indurated edge and a smooth shallow base. The lesion develops slowly over many months and the lymphatic glands are not involved. Squamous carcinoma is more rapid in its growth.

43 Basal cell carcinoma of the hand can be compared with the squamous epithelioma seen in **38**. The edge is not everted and the base is clean.

44 Malignant melanoma This darkly pigmented lesion had been present for only a few months and had grown large in a few weeks. Secondaries developed in the inguinal glands.

45 Malignant melanoma of heel This lesion developed rapidly in an elderly man. Signs of necrosis are present. Note not all malignant melanomas are pigmented.

42

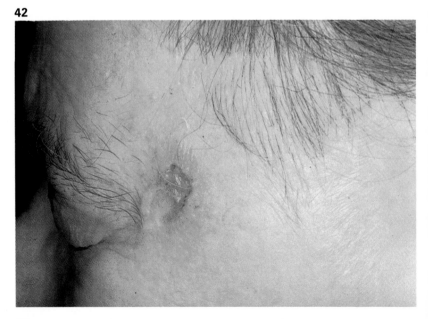

43

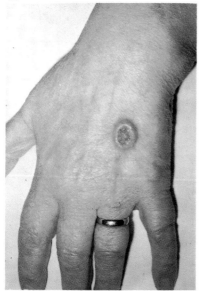

44

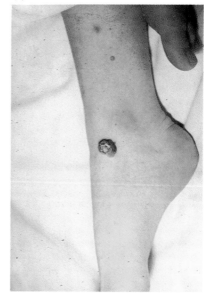

45

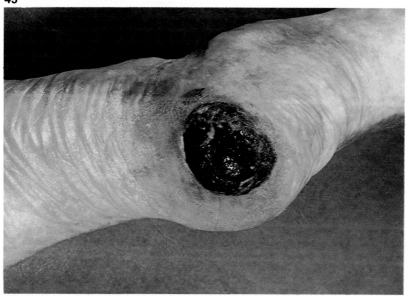

46 Malignant melanoma of big toe This occurred in a 74-year-old man who was thought to have occlusive vascular disease with a gangrenous bleeding patch on big toe. Biopsy was done because the condition did not clear up or extend, and showed presence of malignant melanoma. It should have been remembered that gangrenous areas do not bleed!

47 Malignant melanoma may appear as a bluish area under a nail. The area gradually extends but glands may be enlarged at an early stage and the primary tumour missed unless the nails are inspected as routine.

48 Kaposi's sarcoma (multiple idiopathic haemorrhagic sarcoma) This is a rare lesion, more common in the Eastern Mediterranean and Africa. Multiple purple or brownish nodules appear and develop slowly, in this case in an amputation stump. Diagnosis is confirmed by biopsy.

49 Metastases may occur in the skin anywhere in the body. In this case the secondary is in the umbilicus from an intra-abdominal cancer.

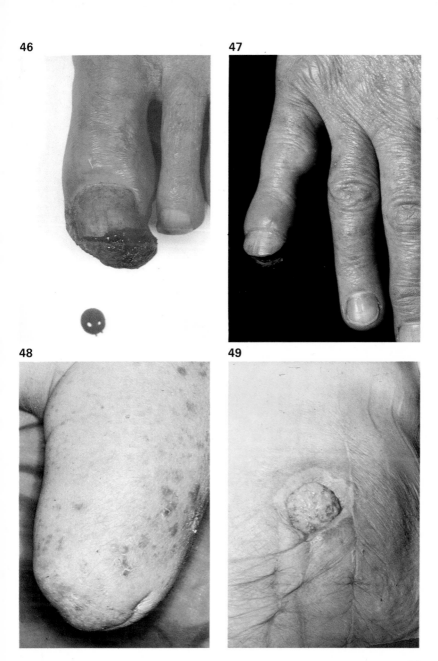

Pre-malignant

50 Bowen's disease This intradermal condition appears as an area of brownish induration with a well defined edge. Keratin crusting occurs. A carcinoma may appear as a nodule or under the crust. It can also be associated with internal carcinoma.

51 Lentigo appears as a flat dark lesion in the cheek of elderly people. It grows slowly and is regarded as a melanoma-in-situ.

52 Malignant lentigo The lesion is frankly malignant with an increase in size of the swelling and increased pigmentation.

53 Solar keratosis Small irregular plaques appear on the skin of the face and hands of fair skinned people especially in the tropics. Some of these warty plaques may turn into carcinoma.

50

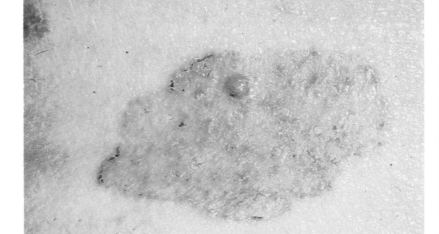

51

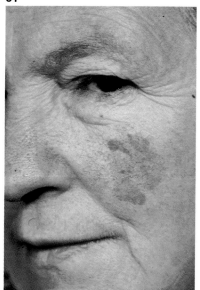

52

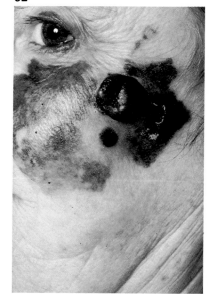

53

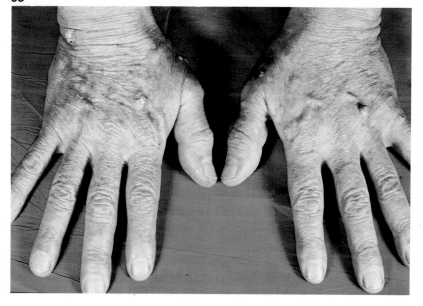

54 Arsenical keratosis This appears usually on the fingers or soles of the feet as multiple corn-like lesions. A history of ingestion of arsenic is obtained.

55 Leucoplakia may occur in the lip, tongue, oral mucosa and vulva. It appears as white thickened patches usually soft but may become enamel-like. A carcinoma is seen developing.

56 Radiodermatitis As in any scarred condition malignancy may develop after many years.

57 Erythema-ab-igne Squamous epithelioma may occur in an area of chronic induration due to exposure to a fire.

54

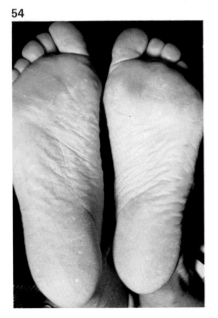

55

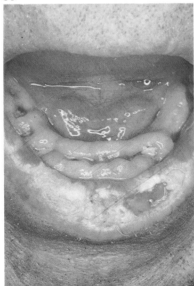

56

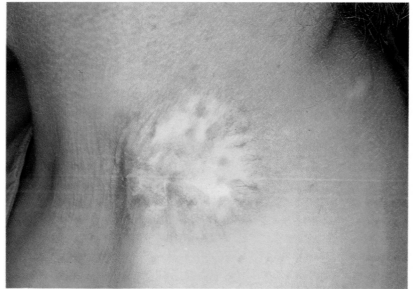

57

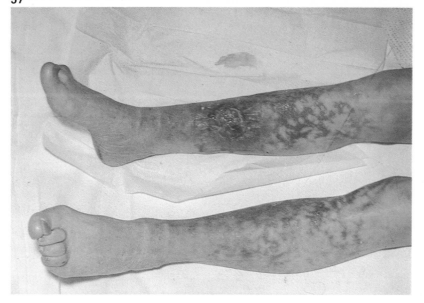

58 Marjolin's ulcer is the development of a squamous epithelioma in a burns scar.

59 Varicose ulcer may, in a few cases, be complicated by the development of a squamous carcinoma.

60 Sebaceous cyst This is not usually thought of as a pre-malignant condition but occasionally as in the lesion behind the ear, a carcinoma may develop. It is sometimes missed if the cyst is not examined histologically.

61 Lupus vulgaris Before the advent of anti-tuberculous therapy this lesion could be very extensive and destructive. Squamous carcinoma could develop in scar tissue.

58

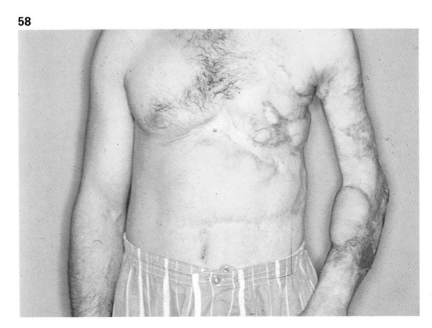

59

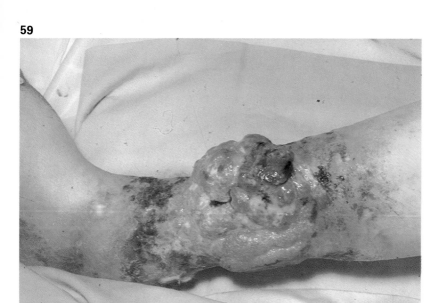

60

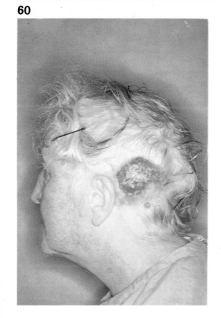

61

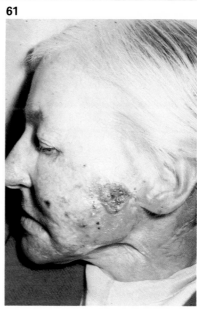

Skin changes in malignancy

62 Acanthosis nigricans There is a darkening of the skin in flexural areas of the body. The dark areas are thickened and rough. Malignancy may be present in the body or develop later. This patient had a carcinoma of colon.

63 Pemphigoid Large bullae erupt on otherwise normal skin and sometimes mucous membrane. Aetiology is unknown. This patient had a cancer of the stomach and after gastrectomy the skin eruption cleared up.

64 Pigmentation of the lips This is usually associated with the Peutz-Jeghers syndrome; i.e. polyps of small intestine, stomach or colon. Normally these polyps are benign. This type of pigmentation has been seen with rectal and colonic carcinoma and with cancer of the pancreas.

65 Dermatomyositis appears as patchy heliotrope coloured markings in face and extremities, especially the malar area of the face.

66 Dermatomyositis of finger Flat topped heliotrope papules over the backs of the finger joints are known as Gottron's sign and are pathognomic of the condition. The incidence of malignant disease varies from 25–50%. Cancer of alimentary canal and lungs are the most common.

62

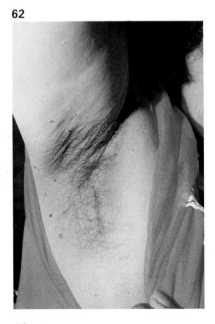

63

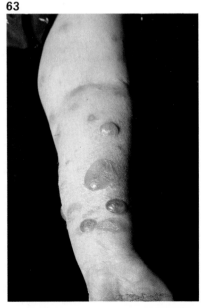

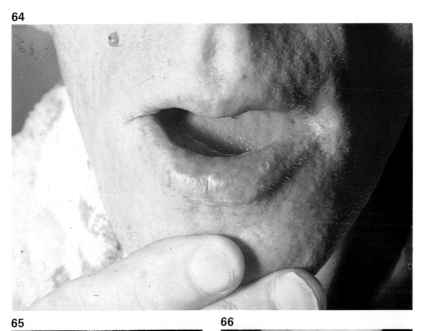

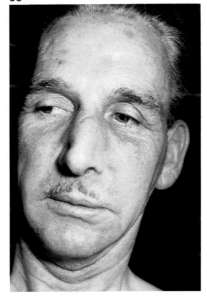

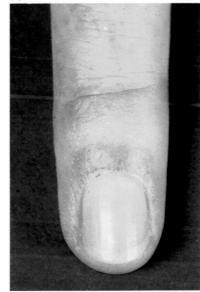

67 Erythroderma is a dry pruritic red change in the skin which is associated with the reticuloses, especially Hodgkin's disease.

68 Erythroderma of the hands There is marked scaling.

69 Carcinoid facies The malar flush is seen with carcinoid tumour of small bowel and is part of the carcinoid syndrome.

70 Herpes zoster There appears to be an increasing incidence of diffuse types of *herpes zoster* with lymphoma and leukaemia especially Hodgkin's disease. This patient had chronic lymphatic leukaemia.

67

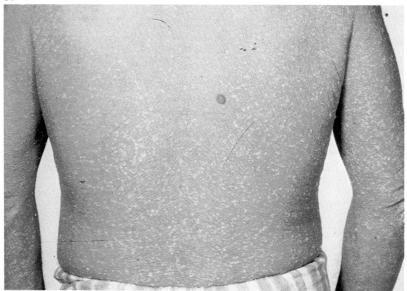

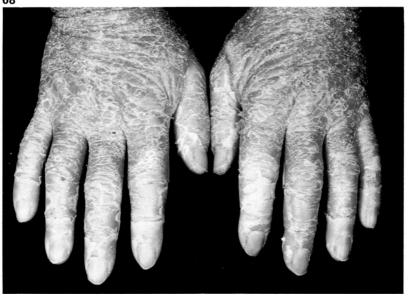

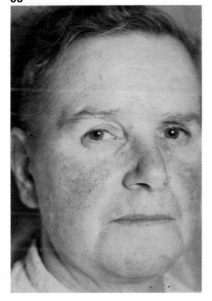

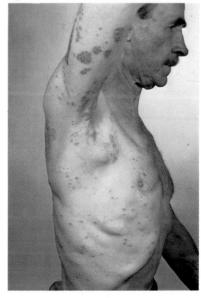

Sinus and Fistula

Sinus

This is defined as a tract lined by granulation tissue between the surface and deeper tissues. The cause of the chronicity of the condition may be a foreign body, infected bone, or chronic abscess cavity. Unresolved infection is the basic underlying cause.

71 Pilonidal sinus The midline of the sacral area is the characteristic site for this common condition. It usually occurs in dark-haired hirsute individuals as dark hairs are harder than fair hairs.

72 Osteomyelitis with sinus The abscess which develops with osteomyelitis may burst externally to effect a connection between skin and infected bone.

73 Dental sinus An apical abscess in upper jaw has burst externally. A probe can be passed down the tract to the root of the tooth. X-ray would show rarefaction around a tooth.

71

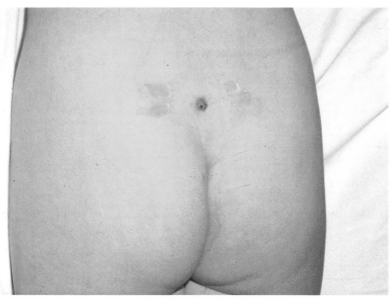

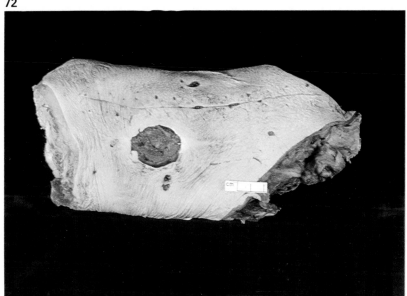

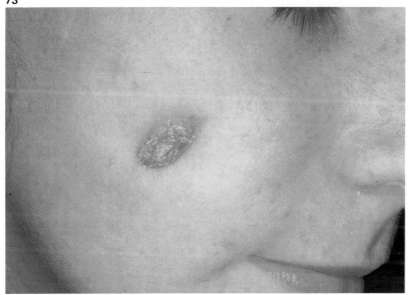

74 Median mental sinus The cause is the same as in **73**. The distance of the sinus opening from the teeth sometimes leads to a mistaken diagnosis. X-ray of the teeth will again show the rarefaction of a tooth root.

75 Median mental sinus The connection between the sinus and responsible tooth can be seen.

76 Abscess with sinus The sinus tract led down to a pericolic abscess. Injection of radiopaque material down the tract showed no connection with the colon.

77 Actinomycosis with sinus The sinus connected with an abscess cavity in the right iliac fossa. 'Sulphur granules' were present in the discharge and microscopy showed presence of the mycelium.

78 Tuberculous sinus in the neck of an elderly man. The sinus led down to caseous glands. Tubercle bacilli were present in the discharge.

74

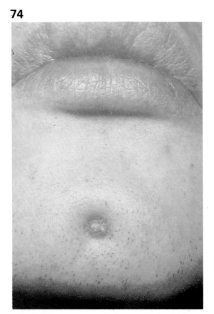

75

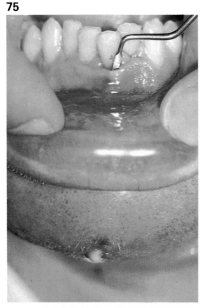

76

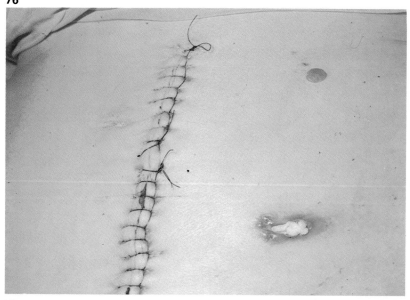

77

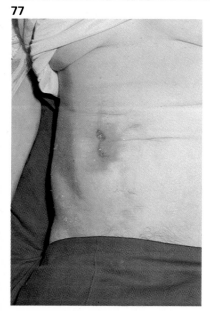

78

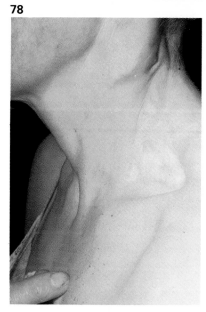

Fistula

A fistula is defined as a tract between two epithelial or endothelium surfaces – skin, mucous membrane, vascular endothelium. It may be external or internal.

79 Branchial fistula nearly always opens in the lower third of the neck at the anterior border of the sternomastoid muscle. Injection of radio-opaque material will show the extent of the fistula.

80 Duodenal fistula This usually follows a partial gastrectomy and opens in the right hypochondrial region. Bile escapes and marked digestion occurs in surrounding skin due to presence of ferments.

81 Ileal fistula related in this case to Crohn's disease. As shown here more than one fistula may be present. Discharge is usually slight and faeculent. Radiography demonstrated connection with the bowel.

82 Ileostomy This may be classified as a fistula except that the bowel is brought up to the skin surface by design as in management of ulcerative colitis, or in creation of an ileal bladder.

79

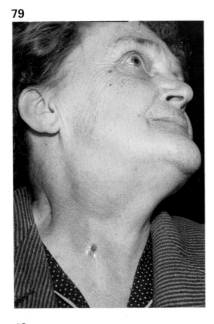

80

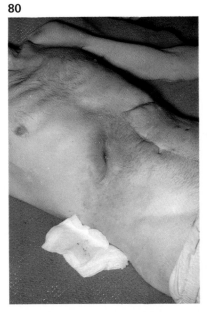

81

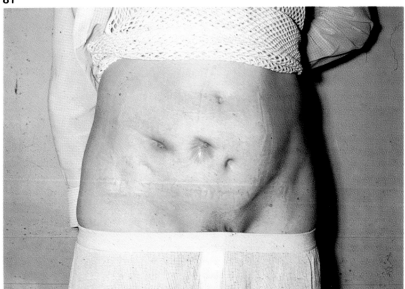

82

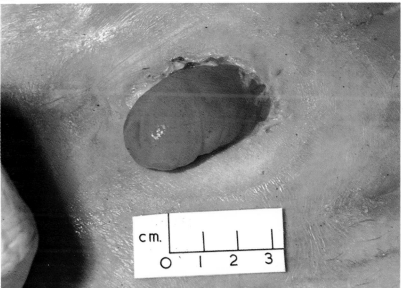

83 Faecal fistula A portion of the terminal ileum has been trapped in a hernia – Richter's hernia. An abscess developed which burst through the skin.

84 A colostomy is a type of faecal fistula where the colon is brought up to the skin surface to relieve pressure in the colon.

85 A caecostomy An opening made between the caecum and skin is another form of faecal fistula. The rubber tube drains the caecum.

86 Extroversion of the bladder is one type of urinary fistula where the urine is discharged on to the skin. It is a congenital lesion.

83

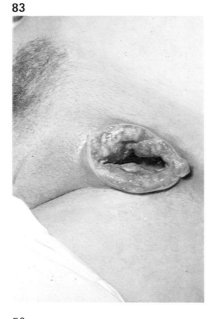

84

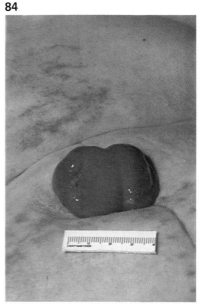

85

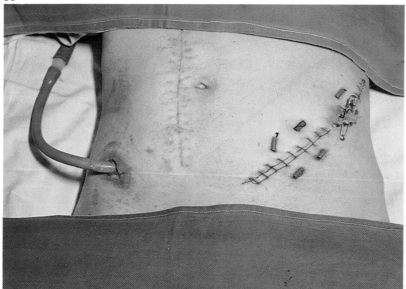

86

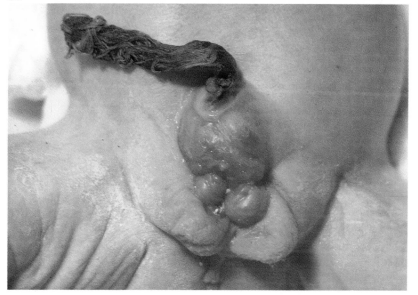

87 Fistula-in-ano connects the rectum with the peri-anal skin. This patient had multiple fistulae due to Crohn's disease of the rectum.

88 Arteriovenous fistula in this patient was present since birth. Unsuccessful operative attempts have been made to excise or block the many connections between arteries and veins.

87

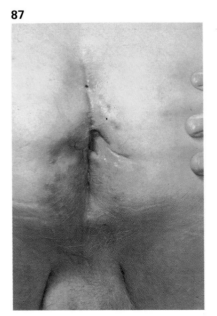

88

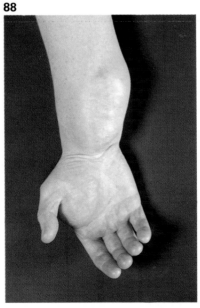

Gangrene

This is defined as death of the tissues. The clinical features depend on the acuteness of onset of the ischaemia and the amount of fluid contained in the tissues.

Clinical features
1 Colour – This varies from early blanching or congestion to final dark brown or black colour. If gas is present patches of brown or green may be seen and blebs may develop.

2 Temperature – Tissue becomes cold and assumes temperatures of the environment. Note false warmth may be present if the limb is artificially heated.

3 Sensation – Ischaemia produces early anaesthesia but this does not necessarily mean tissue death. Although the tissue is insensitive the patient may complain of pain.

4 Function – Muscle power is lost.

Types Dry gangrene usually means a gradual onset in a desiccated limb. Moist gangrene results from ischaemia in a limb or tissue full of blood, i.e. venous obstruction. Infection and action of gas-forming organisms also produce moist gangrene.

Causes of gangrene

Vascular disease
Arteriosclerosis
Thrombo-angiitis obliterans
Raynaud's disease
Diabetic gangrene
Embolism
Thrombosis
Ergot poisoning
Scleroderma
Disseminated intravascular coagulation
Low output failure

Trauma
Cervical rib
Pressure burn
Electrical burn
Frost bite
Trench foot
Pressure gangrene
Tension gangrene
Gas gangrene

89 Typical dry gangrene due to atheroma of lower limb vessels notably affects femoral artery and arteries below the knee.

90 Dry and moist gangrene The little toe shows dry gangrene with infection, and spreading moist gangrene on to plantar surface of the foot. Primary cause was atheroma but infection developed.

91 Combined moist and dry gangrene due to venous and arterial blockage of both legs. The blisters are evident just beyond the dressing which covers more blisters.

92 Raynaud's disease with gangrene of finger due to spasm of the digital artery and thrombosis.

89

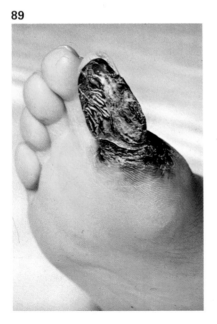

90

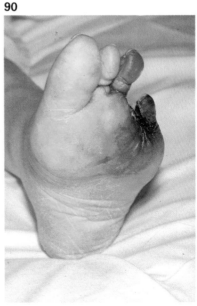

91

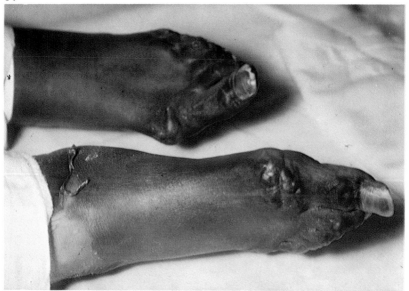

92

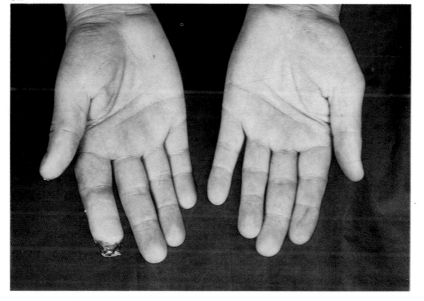

93 Diabetic gangrene is likely to be combined dry and moist due to the infection.

94 Another form of diabetic gangrene is that which occurs in a carbuncle in a diabetic. The central skin became ischaemic due to pressure and infection.

95 Cervical rib can result in gangrene of digits due to emboli showering off from an area of thrombosis in relation to the ribs.

96 Embolism from a clot in left auricle in a patient with mitral stenosis.

97 Thrombosis of the axillary artery with digital gangrene due to a portion of thrombus impacting in the radial and ulnar arteries.

93

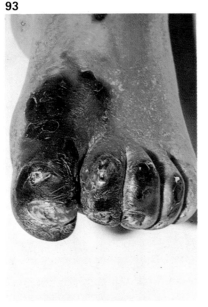

94

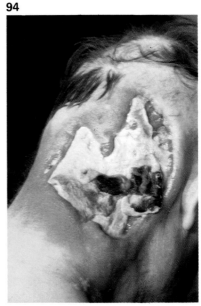

95

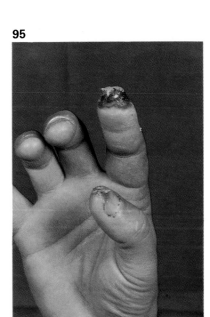

96

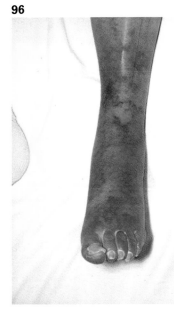

97

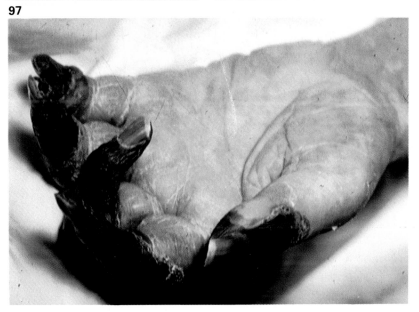

98 Scleroderma of the hands may also result in gangrene due to changes in the smaller arteries and arterioles.

99 Intravascular coagulation associated with shock may produce gangrene as in this patient.

100 Gangrene of the nose caused by low cardiac output. The patient suffered from a coronary thrombosis.

101 Pressure sore This is an example of death of tissue due to ischaemia caused by direct pressure.

98

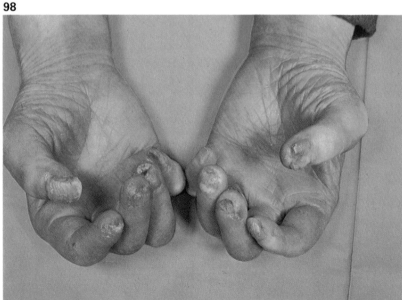

99

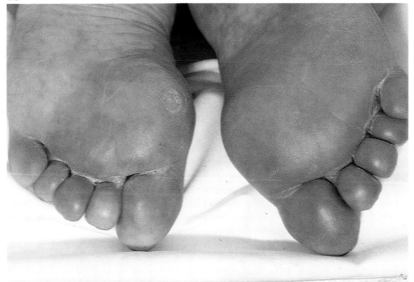

100

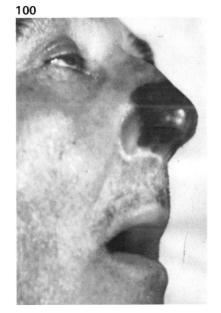

101

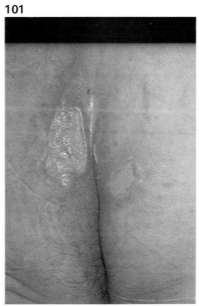

102 Trench foot is the result of the effect of a cold wet environment on the foot. This patient was a soldier in the First World War who had amputations for gangrene.

103 Areas of gangrene on the toes of this baby were caused by cold injury to the foot.

104 Gas gangrene due to a gun-shot wound of buttock contaminated with clostridia.

102

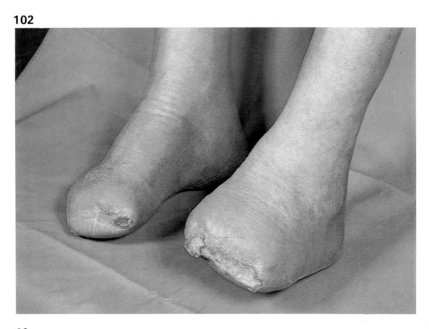

103

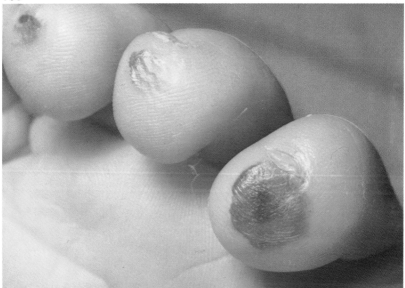

104

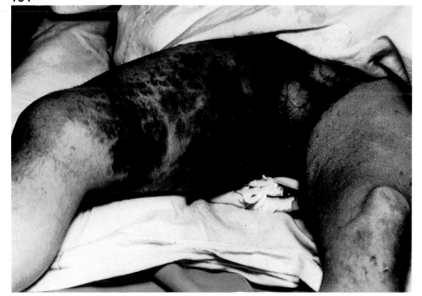

105 The gas produced by the gas gangrene organism can be seen on radiographs of this patient who had gas gangrene of a leg.

106 Gas gangrene due to *Cl. Welchii* infection of abdominal wound. The necrotic skin sloughed off.

107 Pressure gangrene caused by a too tight splint in treatment of a fracture of the forearm.

108 Tension gangrene may occur in an amputation stump where tension on the flaps of an ischaemic limb may be too much for the blood supply.

109 Direct electrical injury to the fingers has caused the gangrene in this typical electrical burn.

105

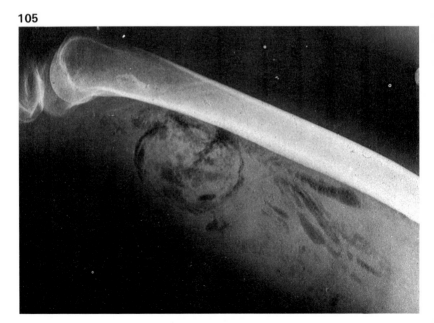

106

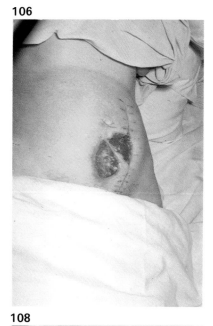

107

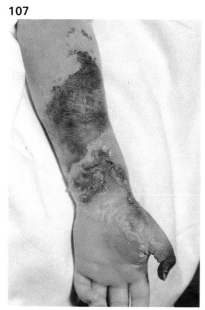

108

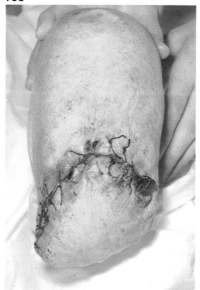

109

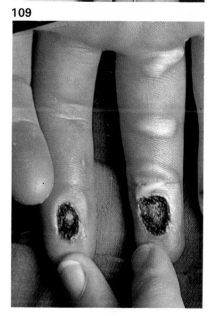

Ulcers

An ulcer is defined as a solution of skin or mucous membrane epithelial tissue. The diagnosis of the type of ulcer is based on the history of its development, clinical examination, and the results of microscopy and or culture.

History Significant facts are: age of patient, trauma, presence of disease – i.e. diabetes, ischaemia, pain, infection, blood dyscrasia, duration and mode of development.

Clinical examination This should elicit the size and shape of the ulcer, whether single or multiple, its progress and the involvement of lymphatic glands. The base or floor and edge of the ulcer, presence of discharge and state of surrounding tissues should be noted.

Classification of ulcers

Traumatic or pyogenic	Due to specific micro-organisms	Malignant ulcer	Special type
Varicose	Syphilis	Rodent	Peptic
Gravitational	Tuberculosis	Epithelioma	
Trophic	Scrofuloderma	Ulceration	
Ischaemic	Soft chancre	Adenocarcinoma	
Pressure	Lupus vulgaris		
Gout	Actinomycosis		
	Tropical ulcer		

Traumatic or pyogenic

110 Varicose ulcer is usually situated on lower half of medial side of the leg above or near the medial malleolus. The base is depressed with granulations and yellowish slough. The edge is irregular, reddened and tender. Enlarged superficial veins are seen.

111 Varicose ulcer On the left leg the ulcer is on the lateral side, the base has a greyish green slough. Surrounding varicose dermatitis and inflammation is marked.

112 Gravitational ulcer results from previous deep vein thrombosis. Oedema of the foot and leg is usually present. The ulcer is as a varicose ulcer but often more extensive than usual. Varicose veins are absent.

113 Trophic ulcers These occur in anaesthetic areas such as sole of the foot in spina bifida, locomotor ataxia etc. In this patient part of the thumb has ulcerated away and practically healed. He had syringomyelia. The ulcers are painless and penetrate towards bone.

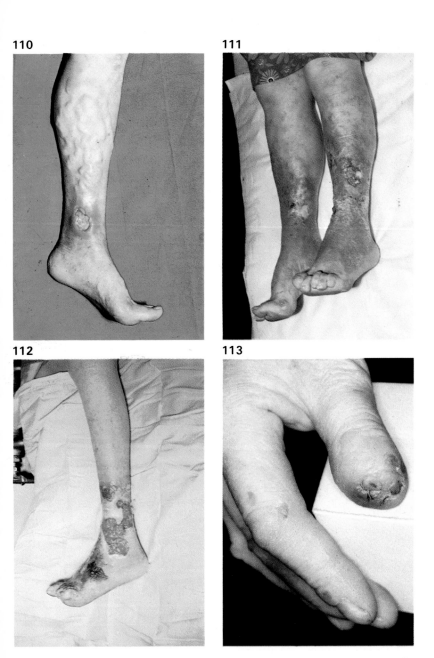

114 Bedsore This large ulcer is in a pressure area in an elderly patient with a fracture of femur. The base is clean but often it is covered with slough and the discharge is offensive. The surrounding skin is shiny and reddened. Pain is not a feature.

115 Bedsore in a paraplegic The ulcers are clean, and they occurred in hospital. The full thickness of the skin is penetrated down to muscle.

116 Pressure sore in the bunion area showing the typical thickened margin of the ulcer extending down to the metatarsophalangeal joint. The ulcer was painful. Patient had occlusive vascular disease with ischaemia.

117 Radionecrosis This is a form of ischaemic ulcer as radiation produces an obliteration of skin vessels. The ulcer has a grey sloughing base with a radiation dermatitis round it.

118 Ischaemic ulcer This occurred in a patient with occlusive arterial disease. The area became reddened then black. When the slough separated tendons were seen in the base. Partial amputation of the foot has resulted.

114

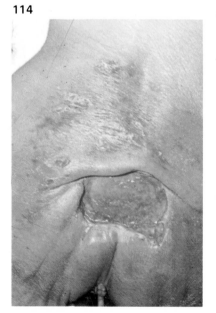

115

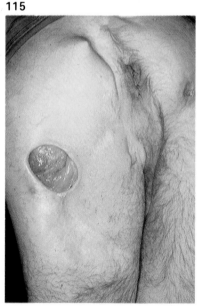

116

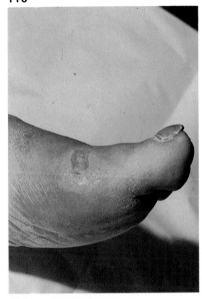

117

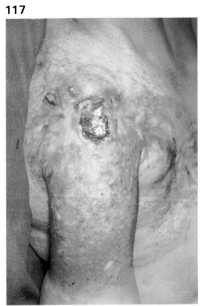

118

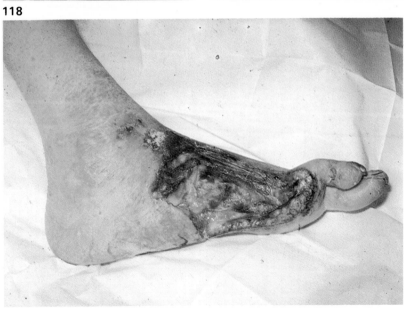

Due to specific micro-organisms

119 Syphilis The syphilitic ulcer shown here in the roof of the mouth has a serpiginous outline. The base has penetrated the palate. A greyish slough is present. The surrounding tissue is healthy. Biopsy was positive.

120 Scrofuloderma This is now a rare condition in which tuberculosis infection has involved the skin and glands with open sinuses, ulcers, and unhealthy skin.

121 Lupus vulgaris In this tuberculosis infection of the skin the ulcers are small and multiple with associated nodules and scarring of the skin. The ulceration can go deeply, with much destruction of soft tissues.

122 Soft chancre of chancroid These appear as multiple ulcers on or near the genitals due to haemophilus ducreyi. The ulcers have a bright red areola with shelving edges and a soft base covered with greenish slough. The lymphatic glands rapidly become enlarged.

119

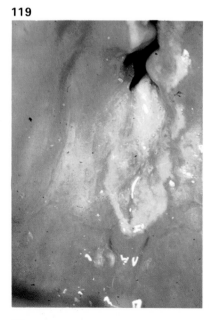

120

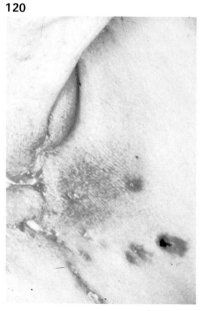

121

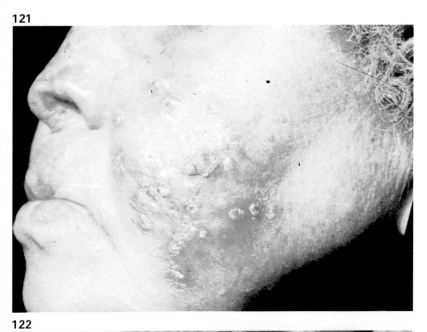

122

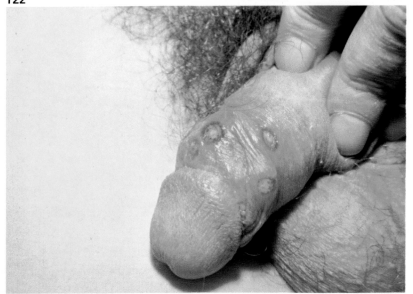

123 Tropical ulcer This is an example of a tropical ulcer seen in Brazil. There are many varieties of tropical ulcer which require examination of the exudate and microscopy to establish the diagnosis.

*(For tuberculosis ulcer see figure **248**.)*

123

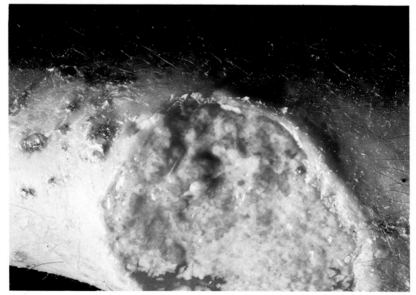

Tissue Tumours

In its broad definition and origin a tumour is merely a swelling. In clinical terms, however, it has become synonymous with the term new growth or neoplasm, and as such it is used in this chapter. Some of the non-neoplastic causes of swellings have been included at the end of this chapter. Diagnosis of tumours is based on history, examination, special investigations and biopsy.

History A number of points in the history are worth emphasising.

1 Congenital – Tumours as apart from swellings are not common at birth. Examples are naevi, which are relatively common, dermoid cysts, cystic hygromas, sacral and coccygeal tumours.

2 Duration – A long history of months to years usually means a benign tumour and a short one of a few months a malignant one.

3 Progress – Rapid growth usually means malignancy. A change in growth rate from slow to rapid may mean malignant changes as in Melanoma.

4 Pain is usually associated with malignant tumours due to infiltration of nerves.

5 Ulceration and bleeding are common in malignant tumours.

Examination It is very helpful for the student to devise a method of examination which will give the maximum information. A useful one involves the 10 S's: site, size, shape, substance, surface, skin over, sensation, surroundings, secondaries, and specific disease.

Classification of tissue tumours

	Benign	**Malignant**
Connective tissue	Lipoma	Liposarcoma
	Fibroma	Fibrosarcoma
	Myxoma	Sarcoma
	Chondroma	Chondrosarcoma
	Osteoma	Osteosarcoma
Muscle	Leiomyoma	Leiomyosarcoma
	Rhabdomyoma	Rhabdomyosarcoma
Blood vessel	Haemangioma	Haemangiosarcoma
	Lymphangioma	Lymphangiosarcoma
Haemopoietic tissue	Lymphoma	Malignant Lymphoma
Nerve tissue	Glioma	Glioblastoma
	Neuroma	Neuroblastoma
	Ganglioneuroma	— — —
Epithelial tissue	Adenoma	Adenocarcinoma
	Papilloma	Papillary carcinoma

Benign tumours

124 A lipoma is usually of ovoid or rounded shape and characteristically feels lobulated on the surface. It has a definite edge and is freely mobile. On gentle compression the lobulation may show through the skin. It occurs throughout the body where fat is, but is commonest in the subcutaneous tissues. This example is in the arm.

125 Lipoma of neck This is quite a common site. In the neck the lipoma may be diffuse i.e. soft, lobulated, adherent to skin but without a definite edge. Sometimes several lipomata may be present and may be painful and tender – Dercum's dolorosa.

126 A lipoma of the axilla demonstrated the lobulation made more distinct on pressure on the skin.

127 Neurofibroma is a small round or ovoid tumour in the course of a peripheral nerve. It can move freely transversely but not in the direction of the nerve. Pressure on it may cause pain and paraesthesia. The example shown is unusually prominent.

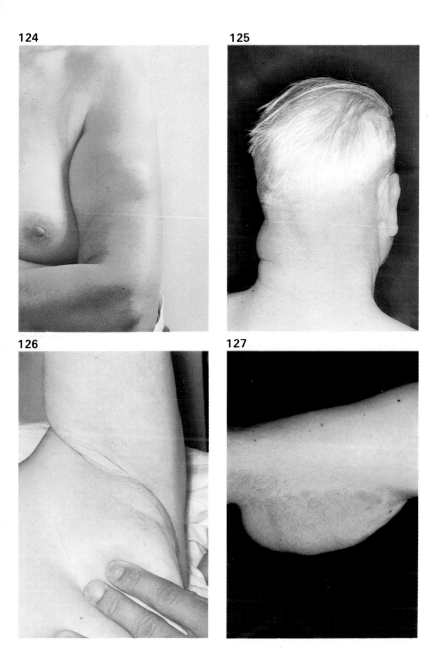

128 Neurofibromatosis (von Recklinghausen's disease) A condition of many neurofibromata scattered throughout the body.

129 Cafe-au-lait spots may be present in the skin especially with the spinal form of neurofibromatosis.

130 A chondroma is a tumour of cartilage. It usually occurs as a slow painless swelling, sometimes multiple, in the hand or foot of young people. It is smooth rounded and firm. X-ray shows a transparent swelling in bone.

131 Osteoma is a benign tumour of bone. This one is from the fontal bone and is very hard.

132 A ganglioneuroma is a rather rare tumour of adult nerve cells and fibres. This example was curious in that it presented as a swelling in the inguinal canal. Diagnosis was made at microscopy.

133 A cut section of 132 showing an amorphous gelatinous appearance.

128

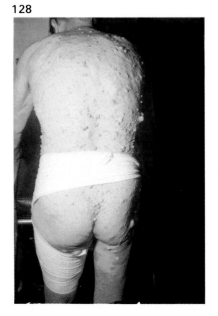

129

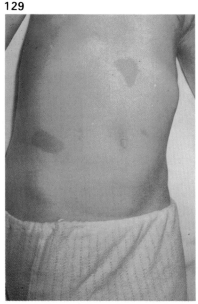

130

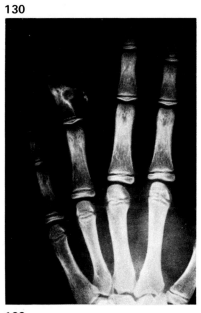

131

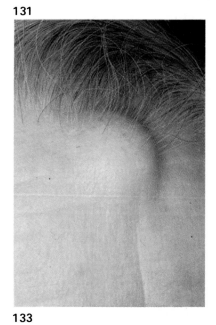

132

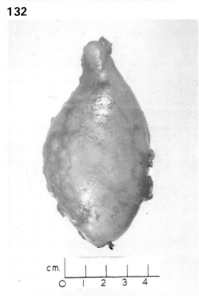

133

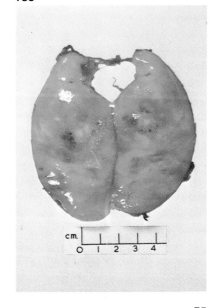

Malignant tumours

134 This liposarcoma of back was much firmer in consistency than a lipoma. It grew rapidly in a few months and was fixed to the surrounding tissues. Diagnosis was made on excision biopsy.

135 A fibrosarcoma was diagnosed on microscopic examination of this rapidly growing, hard and fixed tumour. The back is a common site.

136 A myosarcoma of buttock This appeared as a rapidly growing tumour definitely involving muscle.

137 Sarcococcygeal teratomas are rare but are seen most commonly in infants in the early months of life. There is a typical swelling between the sacrum and rectum. It was firmly attached to the sacrum and coccyx.

134

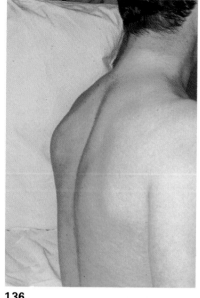

135

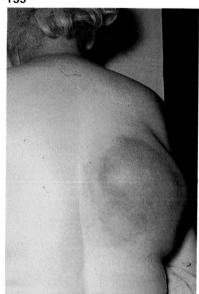

136

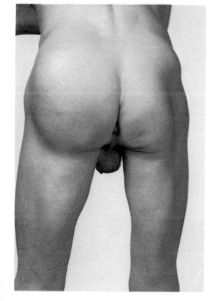

137

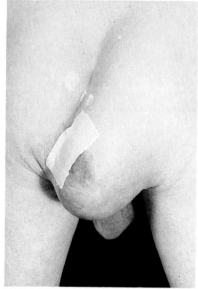

138 Metastatic carcinoma of the arm This looked like a fungating osteogenic sarcoma but the age of the patient was wrong. The primary site was in the bronchus.

139 An osteosarcoma of the upper end of humerus This rapidly growing tumour was diagnosed by x-ray showing typical bone changes and confirmed by open biopsy.

140 A chordoma is a relatively rare tumour that arises from elements of the notochord. The sacrococcygeal region is a known site.

138

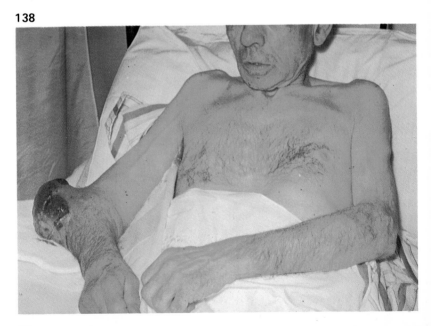

139

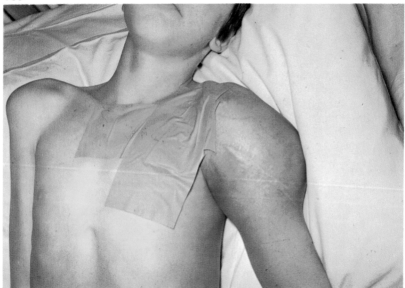

140

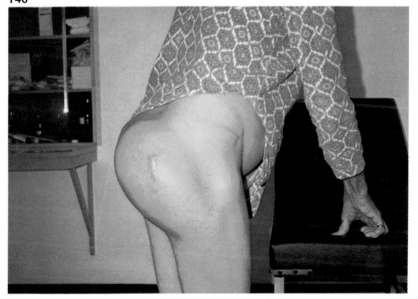

Swellings in tissues

Apart from those due to malformation of limbs, trauma with dislocation or fracture and infection, Swellings may be classified according to their contents:

GAS | *Free* | *Contained*
--- | Emphymsema subcutaneous | In bowel, e.g. hernia
          | Gas gangrene | In lung, e.g. pneumatocoele

Free gas in the tissues gives rise to *crepitus* which is a fine crackling sensation felt by the fingers and the gas is easily displaced by pressure. If a large amount is present it will be tympanitic to percussion. If mixed with fluid as in the bowel a gurgling sound is obtained on pressure.

FLUID | *Water* | *C.S.F.* | *Urine* | *Blood*
--- | Oedema | Encephalocoele | Recognized | Haematoma
           | pits on pressure | Meningocoele | by site and | Aneurysm
           | | occipital | distribution | arterial
           | | spinal | | venous
           | | Spina bifida | |

The main sign of fluid is *fluctuation* which is tested by placing the finger or fingers on one side of the swelling and pressing with the fingers of the other hand on the opposite side. Displacement of the fluid is noticed by the first hand. It should always be repeated in a direction at right angles to the first.

A *fluid thrill* may be elicited in large collections of fluid by placing one hand on the side of the swelling and tapping smartly with the finger on the opposite side.

A sign of transparent fluid is *translucency* when the swelling is grasped firmly to make it tense and a good spotlight is focused on one side with the observer viewing the opposite side possibly through a roll of paper to cut out light passing over the swelling. This sign is used especially in the detection of a hydrocoele.

Blood in the tissues may be in the form of a haematoma which may be firm depending on the amount of clotting present. The skin over it may be bruised or stained with the underlying blood. If the blood is contained in an artery – an aneurysm, a characteristic pulsation will be felt and especially *expansile pulsation* where two fingers on either side of the swelling are bounced upwards and outwards. If the swelling is venous it will be easily compressed and will disappear on elevation of the limb.

141 An encephalocoele is shown with the swelling fixed to the skull. It is somewhat globular in shape, becomes tense on strong expiration, is fluctuant, is sometimes pulsatile and partially reducible into the skull.

142 An occipital meningocoele is similar to **141** but occurs in the occipital region.

141

142

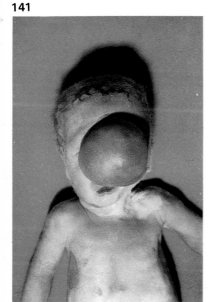
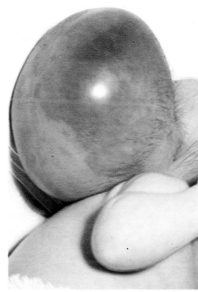

143 A meningocoele is commonly seen in the lumbar region. If it contains nerve elements it is a meningomyelocoele and may then be associated with paralysis of the legs and the bladder.

144 In spina bifida the swelling is in the lumbosacral area and has the characteristics of a meningocoele but is covered by skin. It is tense when the baby cries and is partially reducible within the spine on pressure. On x-ray a defect is seen in the laminae.

143

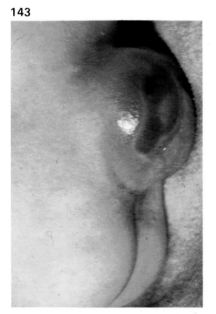

144

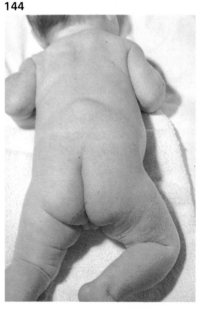

Lesions of the Lips and Face

Lips

145 A hare-lip is an obvious congenital abnormality which should immediately lead to inspection of the palate. It may be unilateral or bilateral and may affect only the lip (simple) or be associated with a cleft maxilla (alveolar type) or with cleft palate (complicated).

146 Obvious flattening of the left nostril with the hare-lip. Inside is a cleft palate.

145

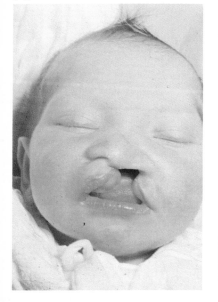

146

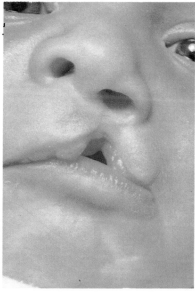

147 A macrocheilia or large lip may be due to a lymphangioma as in this patient in whom the swelling had been present since birth.

148 A cavernous haemangioma of the lip is another rare tumour with a characteristic strawberry appearance. Severe bleeding may occur.

149 A mucous cyst is a common condition. The smooth rounded swelling is topped by a pale almost bluish area where the contained mucus is visible through the thinned mucous membrane.

150 This cutaneous horn has really arisen in the skin at the margin of the lip and involved the mucous membrane.

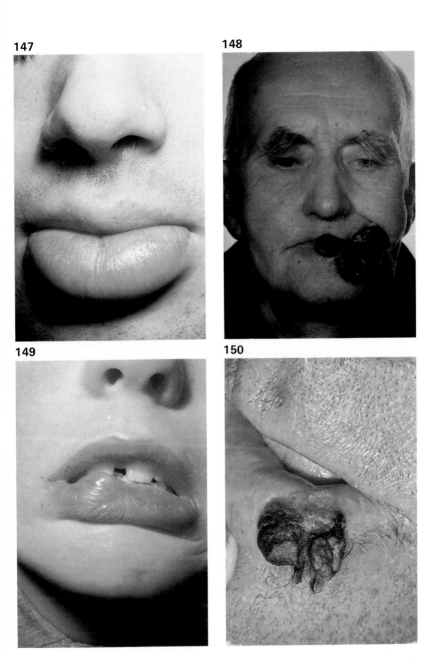

151 A carbuncle may involve the upper lip and the area round the nostrils. The infecting organism was a staphylococcus. The infection may spread along the angular vein to the ophthalmic veins and produce a cavernous sinus thrombosis.

152 Angular stomatitis (cheilitis) due to monilial infection (*candida albicans*) affecting tongue and lips. The white patches are easily scraped off leaving a red surface. This patient was on systemic antibiotics.

MALIGNANT TUMOUR

153 A typical squamous carcinoma of lower lip. The whole area is hard and the edges of the ulcer everted.

154 A squamous carcinoma showing spread to the lymphatic glands on left side of the neck.

151

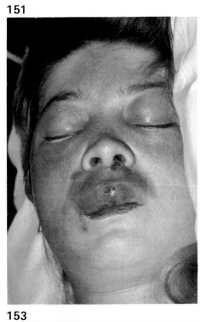

152

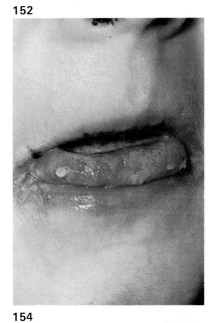

153

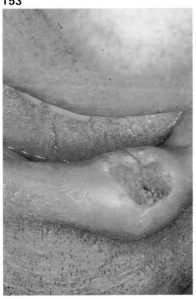

154

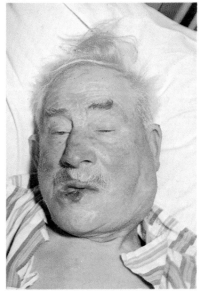

Face

155 Sebaceous cyst appears as a tense rounded, smooth fluctuant swelling. It is fixed to the skin and freely mobile over bone.

156 Rhinophyma This is not really a tumour although it appears as such. It is a hyperplasia of the sebaceous glands on the nose and is common in middle-aged men in whom it is usually associated with rosacea.

157 Cavernous haemangioma of upper lip and nose. The dark compressible lesion full of blood is diagnostic.

158 Cavernous haemangioma of face in the child. The typical strawberry lesion which may clear up in time.

159 Abscess beneath temporal fascia appears as a hot reddened tender swelling above the ear. It is painful and movement of the jaws may be painful. It is within the limits of the temporal fascia.

155

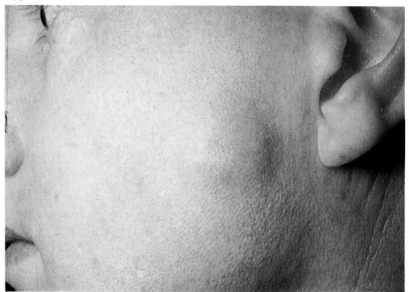

156

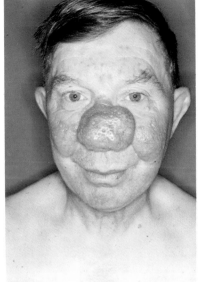

157

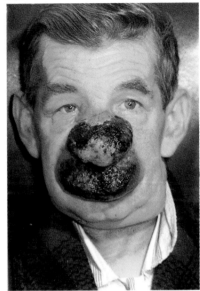

158

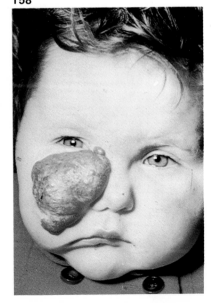

159

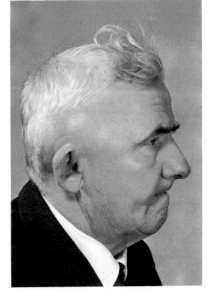

160 Haematoma of face followed on injury but no bruising of the skin was evident as it might have been.

161 Simple melano-naevus of the face of a child. This hairy mole is an intradermal naevus which never becomes malignant.

MALIGNANT TUMOUR

162 Squamous epithelioma involving the ear. The lesion has the typical characteristics of an epithelioma. Secondary glands are present.

163 Basal cell carcinoma of nose. A nodular area with pearly nodules, enlarging slowly with scarring. No glands involved.

164 The typical rodent ulcer in an elderly person. Note the pearly nodules round the central necrotic area.

160

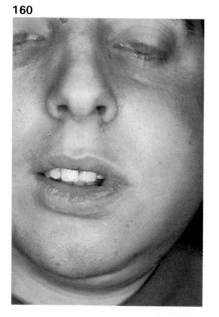

161

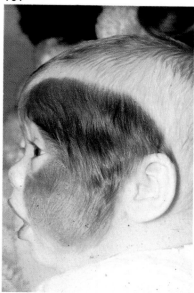

162

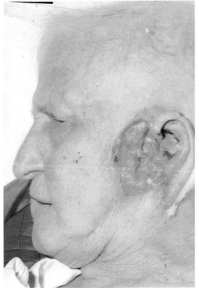

163

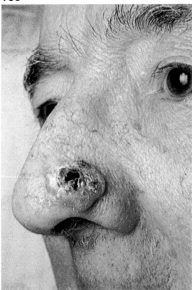

164

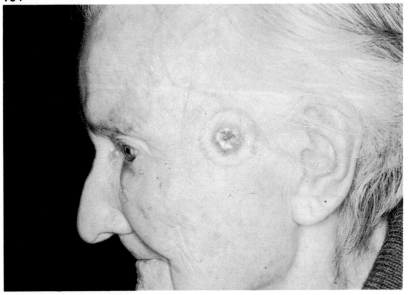

Disease of the Jaws and Orbit

Jaws

ACUTE INFECTION

165 Acute osteomyelitis affecting the maxilla in a baby. An abscess pointing through the hard palate was present. The organism was a staphylococcus. The same was cultured from the mother's nipple.

166 Apical abscess in upper jaw. There was a history of toothache followed by a painful tender nodule. A radiograph showed a lesion at the root of the tooth.

BENIGN SWELLING

167 Masseteric hypertrophy affecting the left masseteric muscle. The aetiology is unknown. Sometimes it is bilateral.

168 Adamantinoma of lower jaw is an example of an odontome, an epithelial tumour arising in dental tissue. X-ray showed the typical soap bubble appearance.

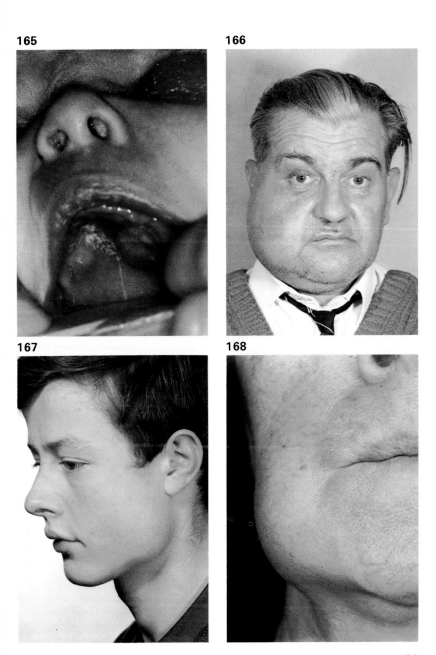

MALIGNANT TUMOUR

169 Carcinoma of left maxillary antrum presents with pain in left side of face and in upper teeth. The left labial fold is absent. Epistaxis may occur. Finally swelling, x-ray evidence and biopsy confirm diagnosis.

170 The swelling of the left maxillary antral carcinoma is more apparent when viewed from above.

169

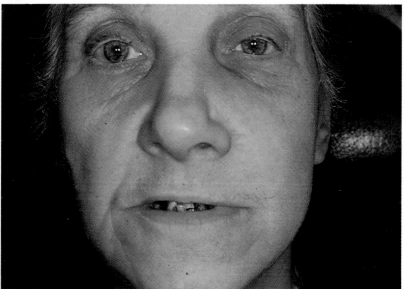

170

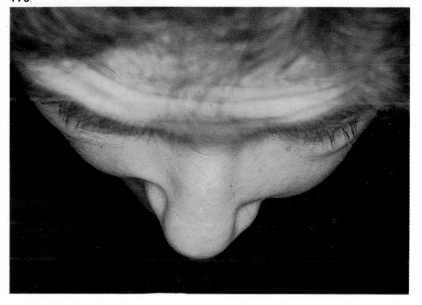

171 Osteogenic sarcoma of the maxilla The swelling is fairly rapid, though pain is not an early feature. Diagnosis by x-ray. This condition is more common in women.

172 A sarcoma of the ethmoid in the patient extended down to involve the maxilla. The appearance is described as the 'frog faced man'.

173 A lymphosarcoma arising in the nasopharynx may spread, as here, to involve the maxilla.

171

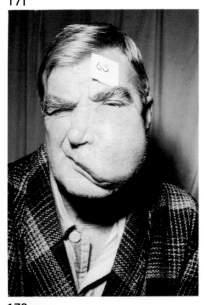

172

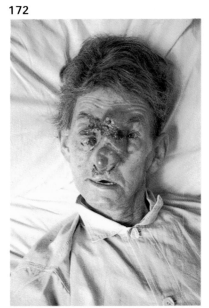

173

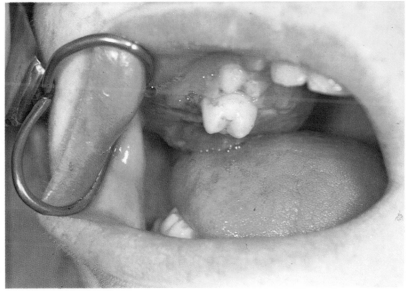

Orbit

INFECTION

174 Orbital cellulitis In this case the infection spread up from the maxilla.

175 Meibomian cyst is due to retention of secretion in the meibomian glands. Infection can occur.

176 Dermoid cyst occurring typically at the lateral end of the left eyebrow is sometimes called an external angular dermoid.

177 Mucocoele of lachrymal gland produces a soft swelling at the inner canthus.

178 The mucocoele is made more prominent by pressure.

174

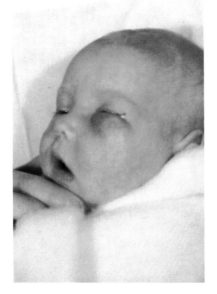

175

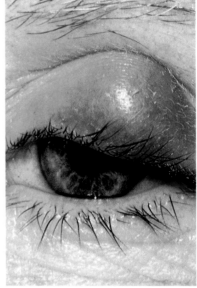

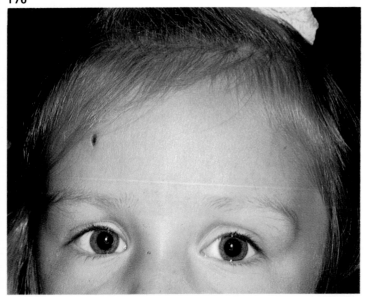

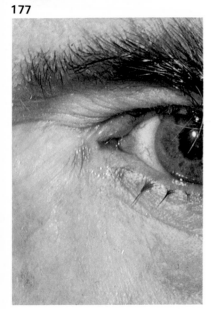

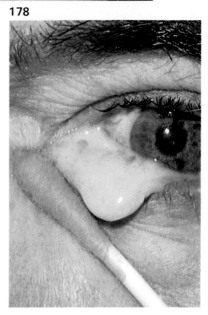

MALIGNANT TUMOUR – EXTRAOCULAR

179 Carcinoma of lachrymal gland appears as a tumour in the inner canthus. The example is a tumour of the lachrymal sac. Biopsy revealed it as a carcinoma.

180 Glioma This involved the right optic nerve producing a proptosis.

181 On proptosis, due to a retro-ocular lesion, the eye is pushed forward with the upper lid in advance, the lower eyelid moves forward and downward.

182 The proptosis is especially noticeable in a lateral view. Some idea of the site of the causative lesion may be obtained from carefully observing the effects on the eye.

183 Invasion of orbit by sarcoma of ethmoid. The expansion of the root of the nose and the discharge through the nostrils suggest origin in the ethmoid. Confirmed by x-ray.

179

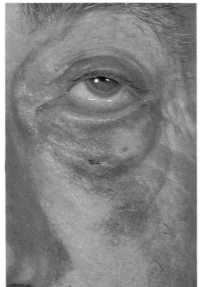

180

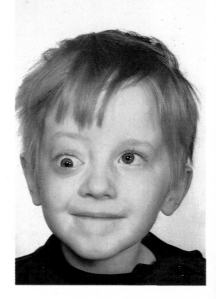

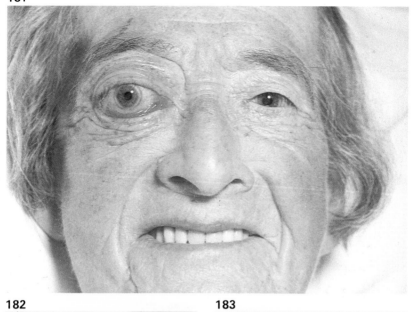

181

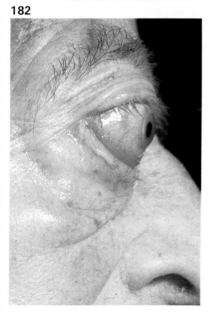

182

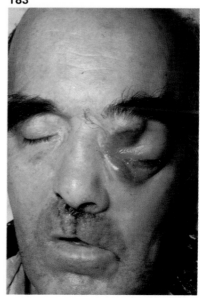

183

184 A secondary tumour from a thyroid cancer producing a slight swelling in upper orbital margin on patient's left side and slight ptosis of left upper eyelid.

MALIGNANT – INTRAOCULAR

185 Retinoblastoma produces a dilated pupil and a curious opaqueness in the eye. Proptosis and blindness occur.

186 Retinoblastoma Examination of the retina shows the tumour.

184

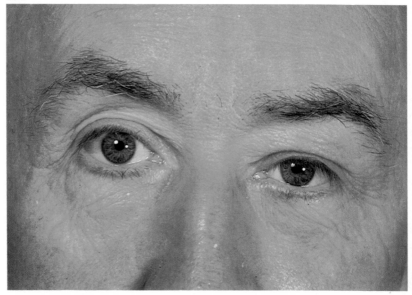

185

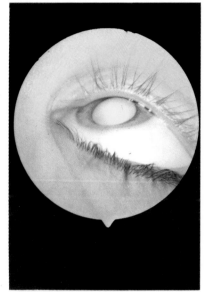

186

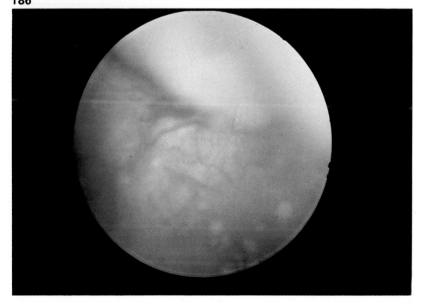

187 Melanoma of the eye is usually seen in the middle aged. A visual defect is noted first. Secondary spread may occur easily. The tumour is visualised on retinoscopy.

188 Lymphoma of upper eyelid is seen as a tumour of the eyelid. Diagnosis is made by biopsy.

MISCELLANEOUS CONDITION

189 Xanthelasma showing the raised yellowish nodules in the skin. They are associated with similar lesions elsewhere and are commoner in diabetics.

187

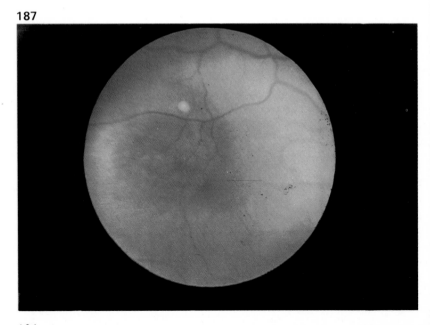

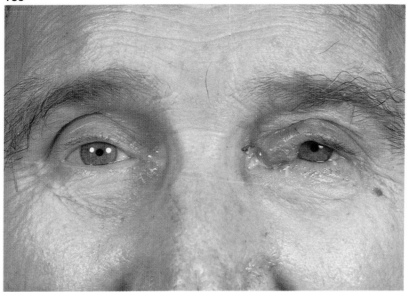

188

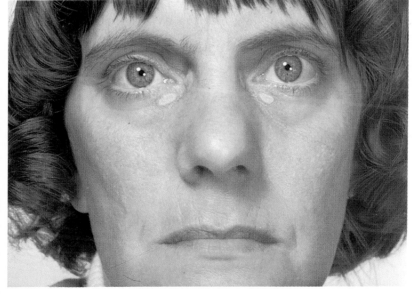

189

Lesions of Salivary Glands

Parotid

Swellings of the gland are bounded above by the zygomatic arch, below by the angle of the mandible, behind is the anterior border of the sternomastoid muscle. They extend forward over the masseter.

INFLAMMATORY LESION

190 Acute parotitis is not common now. It was seen in old patients debilitated by disease and dehydrated. Pain can be considerable, especially on mastication. The area is very tender and red. Bilateral parotitis, especially in young, is probably due to mumps.

191 Parotitis On inspecting the mouth, pus may be seen coming from Stenson's duct.

192 Parotid abscess is suspected if there is increasing pain and tenderness with marked oedema and possibly rigors. Fluctuation is late because of tight overlying fascia. The abscess has been incised with release of pus.

193 Chronic parotitis is commoner in children and young adults. There is recurrent swelling of the parotid. Purulent saliva may be expressed from the duct. Diagnosis is confirmed by x-ray which shows presence of dilated ducts – sialectasis. A narrowing of the main duct is present.

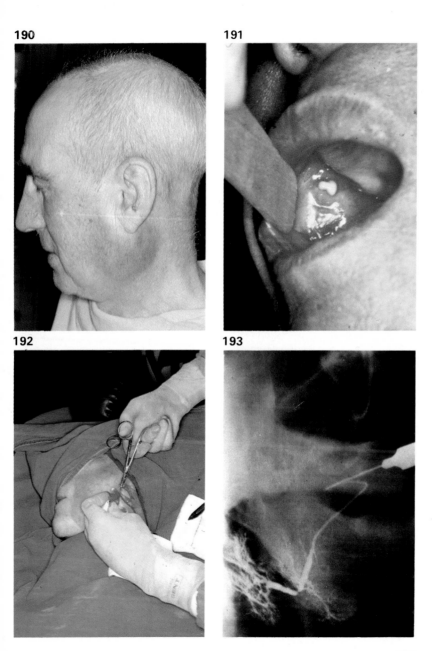

Tumours of the parotid may be classified into three grades: **benign** –
adenolymphoma; **potentially malignant** – mixed parotid tumours;
malignant – carcinoma.

BENIGN TUMOUR

194 An adenolymphoma occurs usually below the lobe of the ear and
behind the angle of the mandible. It is slow growing, commoner in neck, and
characterised by being softer than the other parotid tumours with a cystic
feel.

194

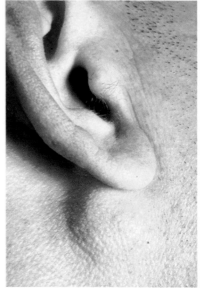

POTENTIALLY MALIGNANT

195 A mixed parotid tumour is the commonest tumour of the parotid gland. It occurs at the same site as the adenolymphoma but is firmer to the touch. It is slow growing and can reach a considerable size.

196 A mixed cell tumour present for ten years. There was no pain or discomfort except for its size.

195

196

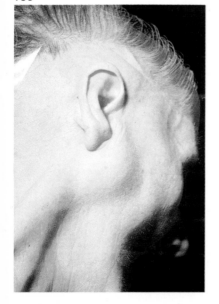
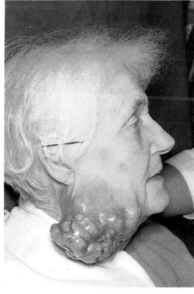

MALIGNANT TUMOUR

197 The mixed tumour may become malignant after a variable time of months to years. It involves the neck and may cause a facial nerve paralysis or may quickly increase in size with danger of ulceration.

198 Carcinoma of the parotid often occurs in the upper part of the gland growing quickly and involving most of the gland. It is hard in consistency.

199 Carcinoma of parotid has extended to affect the facial nerve producing paralysis. Pain in the ear and side of the head and difficulty in opening the mouth are characteristic.

200 Facial nerve palsy on right side due to recurrence of a carcinoma of the parotid excised seven months previously. Sometimes occurs as a post-operative paralysis.

197

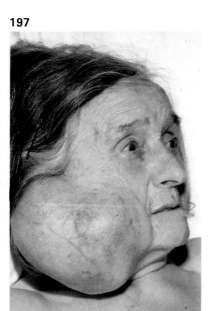

198

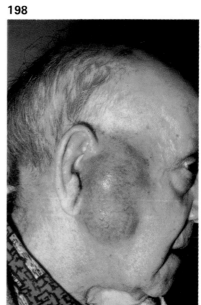

199

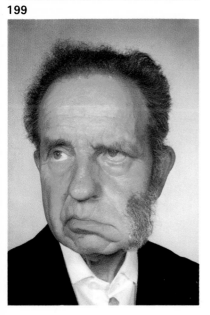

200

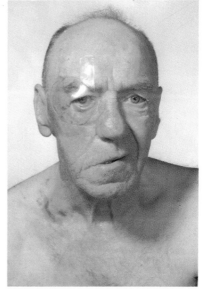

201 This apparent parotid tumour was in fact a lipoma overlying the gland. It had the characteristic soft lobular feel of the lipoma and lay in the subcutaneous tissues.

202 A further diagnostic problem This swelling thought to be a parotid tumour was an abscess in the lymphatic gland overlying the parotid. Its superficial nature and softness suggested the diagnosis confirmed at operation.

201

202

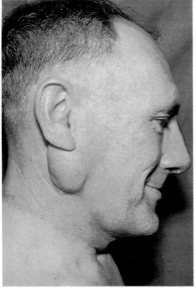

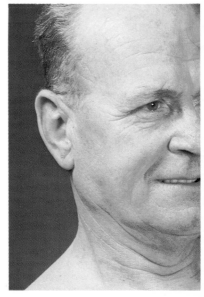

Submandibular salivary gland

203 A submandibular gland abscess may extend backwards in the neck producing a diffuse inflammation over a wide area.

204 Recurrent swelling of the right submandibular gland This is especially noticed during meals. Usually due to a stone in the gland or in Wharton's duct which can be palpated through the mouth.

203

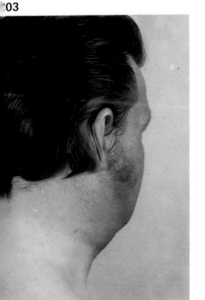

204

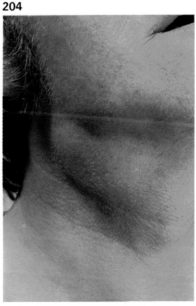

205 Enlargement of the right submandibular duct is evident on inspection as is the pus exuding from the orifice of the duct.

206 Sialogram shows the presence of a stone, previously visible on plain x-ray, in the line of a duct.

207 A stone removed from a submandibular gland.

205

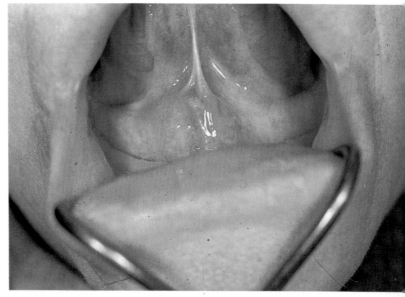

206

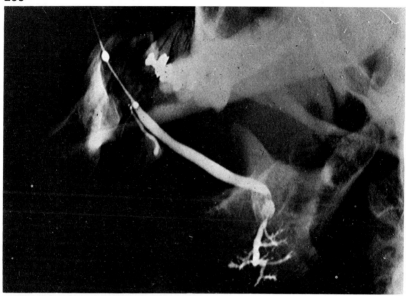

207

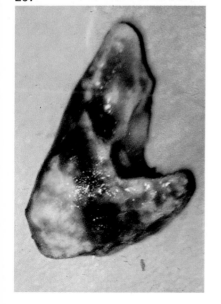

TUMOURS

208 Mixed tumours of the submandibular gland are not common. They are slow growing swellings not affected by taking of food and are firm in consistence.

209 A carcinoma of the submandibular gland appears similar to a mixed tumour except that it grows more readily and will infiltrate the tissues of the neck.

210 Carcinoma in ectopic salivary tissue in the hard palate. This is the most common site, although it may be found elsewhere in the mouth.

208

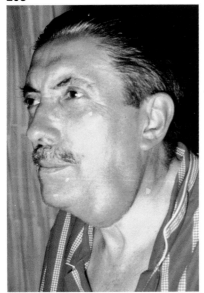

209

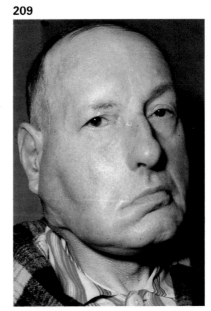

210

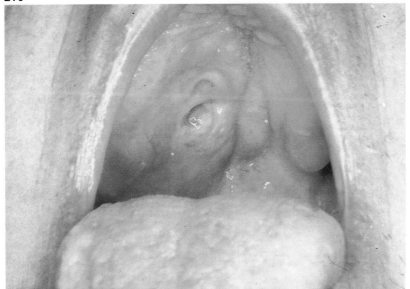

Lesions of Palate and Mouth

Palate

211 Congenital cleft of soft palate.

212 Congenital complete cleft of palate, pre-maxilla and hare-lip.

213 Pyogenic granuloma of hard palate. This arose in relation to a peri-apical infection with root abscess.

214 Monilial infection of gum and palate.

211

212

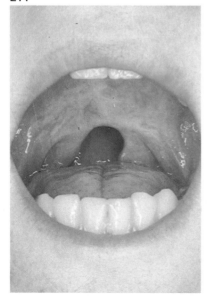
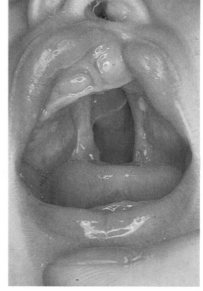

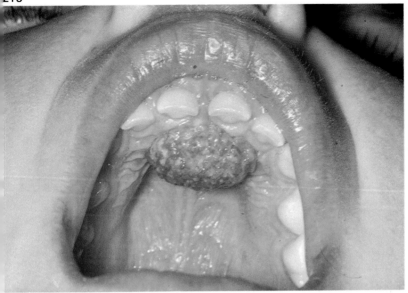

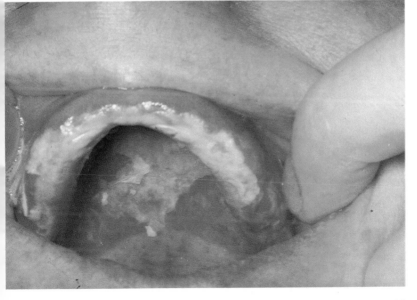

215 Allergic reaction due to dental plate. The reddened granulomatous area is the contact area of the dental plate.

216 Dermoid cyst of palate is seen in the midline. It was incised with release of sebaceous material.

217 Dermoid cyst incised and hair removed.

218 Dental cyst bulging through one side of the hard palate. All the teeth are present on the left side. The cyst arose from the root of a chronically infected tooth. X-ray confirmed the cystic expansion of the alveolus.

215

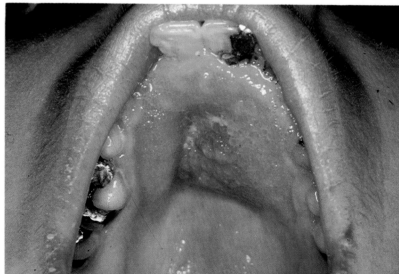

216

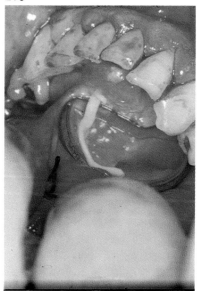

217

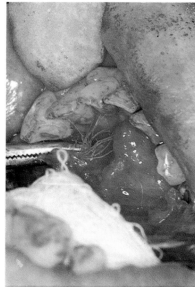

218

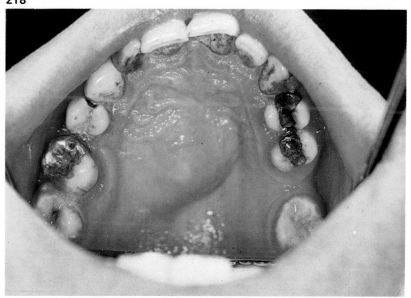

219 Syphilitic perforation of the hard palate is seen in the midline in a tertiary stage of the disease. Wassermann reaction was positive.

220 Adenoma of palate usually appears at the junction of hard and soft palate. It is firm to touch. This one was placed more anteriorly than usual.

221 Epithelioma of hard palate The ulcerated area is typically malignant with sloughing base and everted raised edge.

219

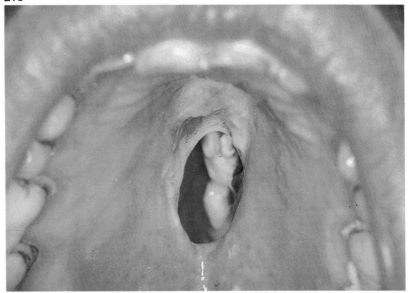

220

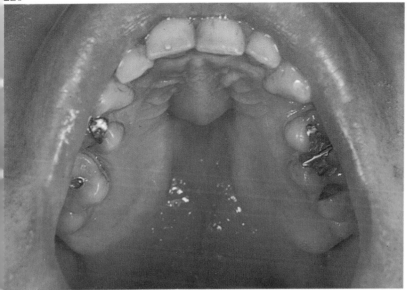

221

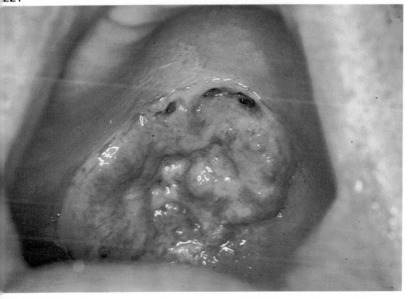

Mouth

222 A sublingual dermoid characteristically presents in the midline of the floor of the mouth on each side of the frenum of the tongue. It is cystic, and the mucosa over it is pink.

223 A rannula in contrast to the above is a cystic swelling on one side of the mouth. As the contents are light coloured the cyst has a bluish sheen.

224 Addison's disease with typical brownish pigmentation of the gums. Sometimes the pigmentation is quite discrete and easy to miss.

222

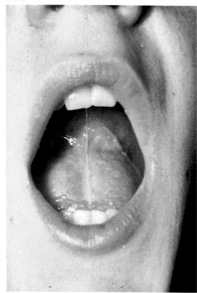

223

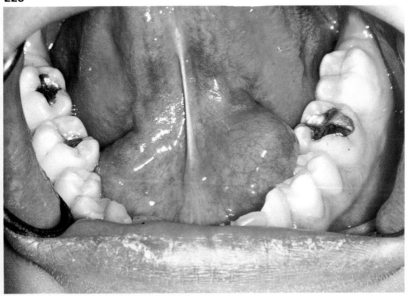

224

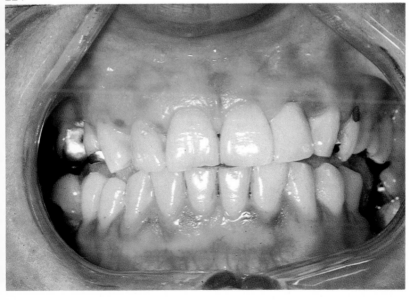

225 Hyperplasia of the gums due to Epanutin therapy.

226 A pyogenic granuloma This occurred in a pregnant woman and disappeared on termination of the pregnancy. Sometimes known as the pregnancy tumour.

227 A myeloid epulis or giant cell granuloma occurs at the gingival margin between two teeth. It grows rapidly as a soft irregular purple mass which bleeds easily.

225

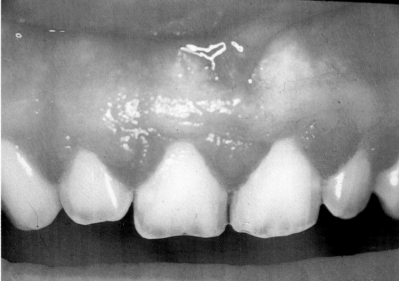

226

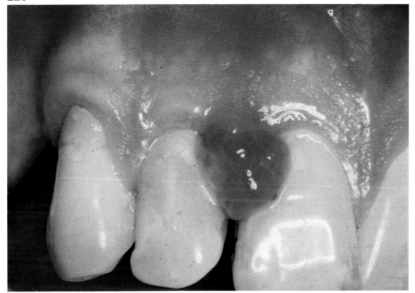

227

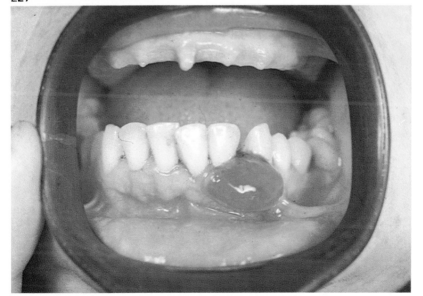

228 This dental cyst arose at the root of the upper right lateral incisor. The bluish buccal expansion is typical. It is at first hard; later 'eggshell crackling' is detected.

229 Ossifying fibroma This is a rare tumour and usually sited in the wall of the maxillary antrum in the subperiosteal region. It grows slowly over the years and is painless. X-ray will show calcification. Biopsy is helpful.

230 Endosteal osteoclastoma The tumour nearly always anterior to the first molar tooth. It tends to become pendunculated and has a short thick stalk. Pain is not a feature of this type. X-ray is unhelpful; biopsy is.

231 Mixed salivary tumour arising in ectopic salivary tissue in the cheek. Biopsy necessary for diagnosis.

232 Squamous epithelioma of alveolus The ulcerating mass is typical of neoplasm.

228

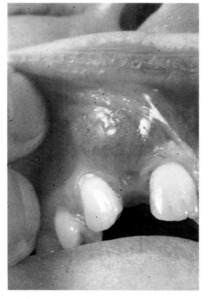

229

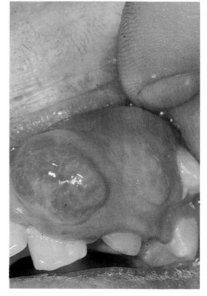

230

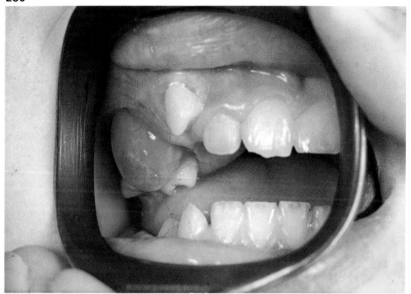

231

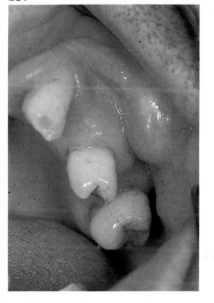

232

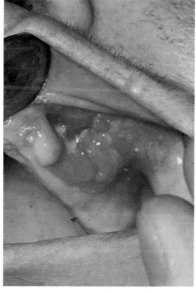

Lesions of Tongue

Congenital, inflammatory, and miscellaneous lesions

233 Tongue-tie The tongue is tethered to the floor of the mouth by a shortened frenum. The patient cannot extend the tip of the tongue beyond the front teeth. There are no symptoms but for appearance sake it is easy to cut the frenum and mobilise the tongue.

234 Acute glossitis The tongue is swollen, oedematous and reddened. The condition improved with Vitamin B.

235 Acute glossitis of milder degree Cause unknown.

236 Erythema multiforme may produce an inflammatory enlargement of the tongue. It may be associated with ulceration of the mouth, eyes, nose and genital orifices. It responds well to steroids.

233

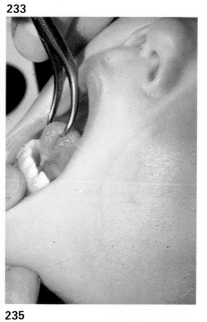

234

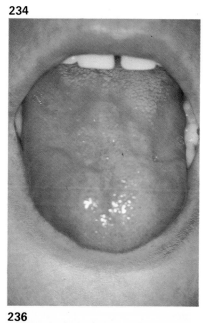

235

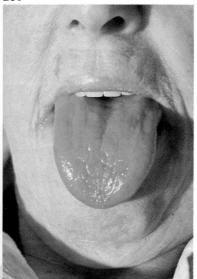

236

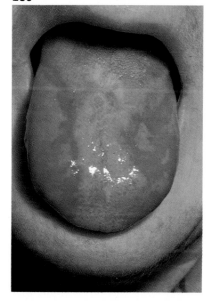

237 Median rhombic glossitis The rhomboid reddened area is situated at the site of the tuberculum impar, and is due to failure of the lateral halves of the tongue to fuse posteriorly. Biopsy will exclude a more serious lesion if in doubt.

238 Pyogenic granuloma This curious reddened swelling was found on biopsy to contain non-specific granulation tissue. It cleared up without treatment.

239 'Raw beef' tongue as described in pernicious anaemia. The red surface is smooth with absence of the filiform papillae. The patient's skin is typical.

240 Telangiectasis in the tongue is an uncommon condition. The red spots are in a variety of areas and are of little clinical significance.

241 Purpura of the tongue The tongue is a rare site of purpura.

237

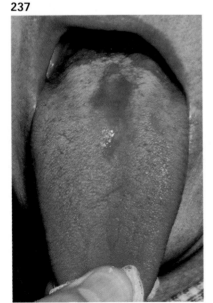

238

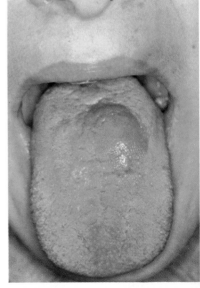

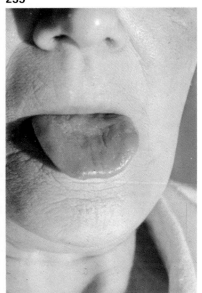

239

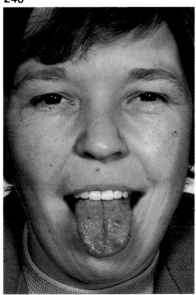

240

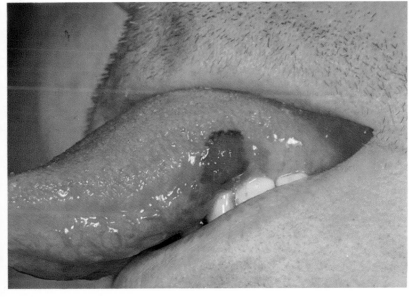

241

242 Atrophy of right side of the tongue due to hypoglossal nerve paralysis. The tongue deviates to the side of the lesion. The nerve was involved in cervical metastases.

242

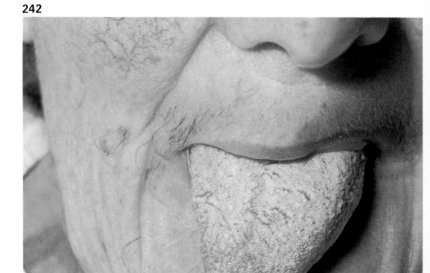

Ulcers in the tongue

243 Herpes zoster may affect one side of the tongue which is covered with typical herpetic lesions. These may ulcerate to leave tiny ulcers.

244 Aphthous ulcer, on the side of the tongue begins as thickening which breaks down in about 24 hours to form a small punched out ulcer with a raised rampant like red margin. It is quite painful.

243

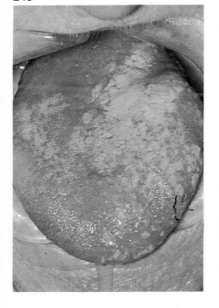

244

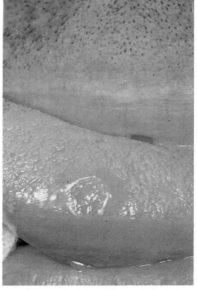

245 Dental ulcer occurs at the side of the tongue opposite a ragged tooth or denture. The presence of a cause confirms the diagnosis. In this case the cause was thought to be due to an electrical discharge from a gold filling.

246 Erosive lichen planus produces a widespread lacy type erythema with superficial irregular ulceration.

247 Chronic non-specific ulcer This chronic, relatively painless ulcer had no obvious cause and was thought might be malignant. Excision biopsy revealed its benign nature.

245

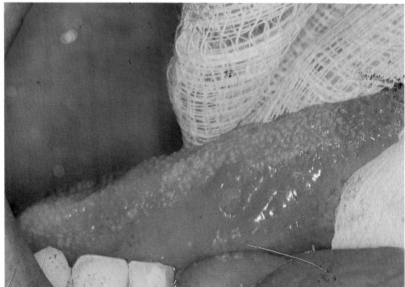

246

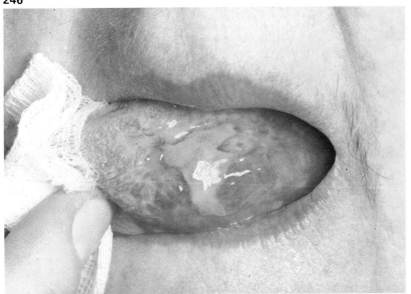

247

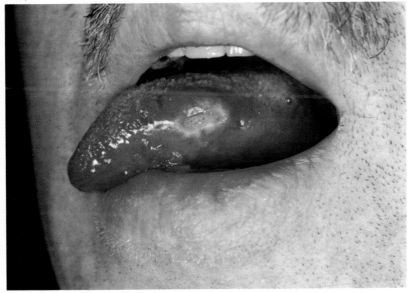

248 Tuberculous ulcer is said to occur most often at the tip or posterior third of the tongue. The patient's sputum was positive for tubercle bacilli.

249 Leucoplakia appears as enamel-like covering of the tongue. Ulceration and bleeding may occur and, if so, suggest malignancy.

250 Leucoplakia The toluidine blue test is said to indicate malignancy. This was certainly true in this case.

248

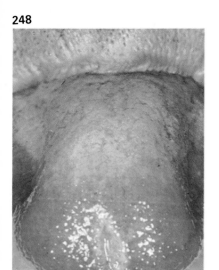

249

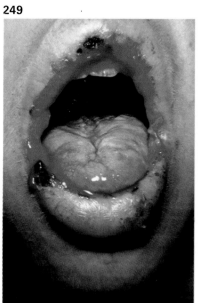

250

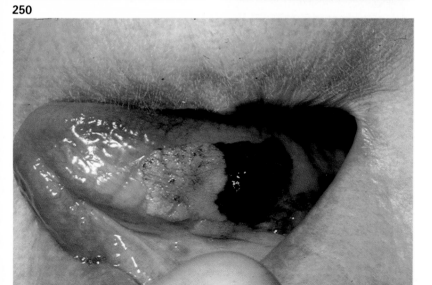

139

Tumours of tongue

BENIGN

251 Angioma of the tongue may be a venous angioma or a lymphangioma. Although the venous type is usually localised and the other produces a macroglossia, biopsy is necessary to establish diagnosis.

252 A papilloma is the most common benign tumour of tongue.

251

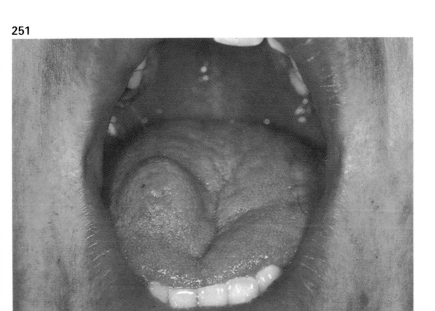

252

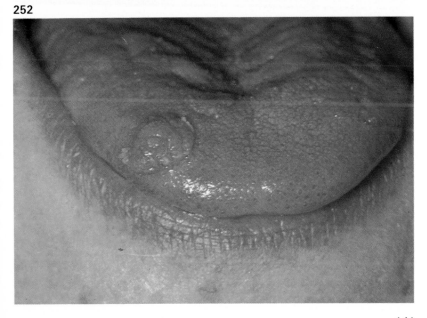

141

MALIGNANT

253 Epithelioma usually occurs at the edge or margin of the tongue and may extend on to the floor of the mouth, or vice versa.

254 Epithelioma may also occur in an area of leucoplakia.

255 After radiation therapy both epithelioma and leucoplakia disappeared.

253

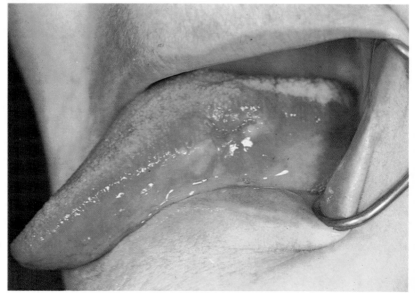

254

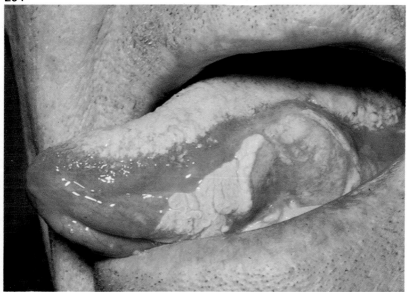

255

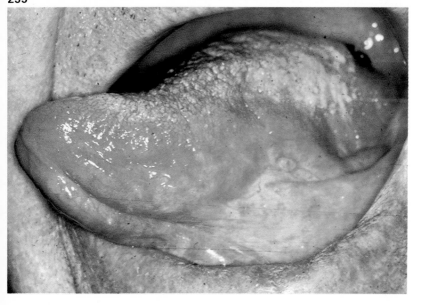

Disease of the Tonsils, Pharynx, Larynx

Tonsils

256 Acute tonsillitis with gross swelling and redness of the tonsils. Thick pus exuding. Children may not complain of much pain.

257 Vincent's infection of tonsil The grey sloughing areas look almost like a malignant tumour, however the whole throat is red and inflamed. Vincent's organisms were prolific.

258 Carcinoma of left tonsil extending up into the palate. Lymph glands in neck were enlarged.

256

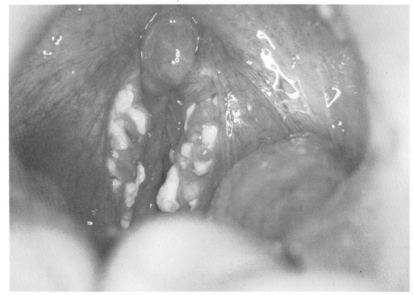

257

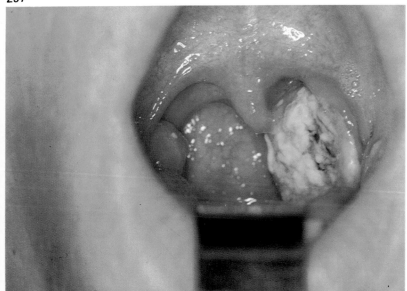

258

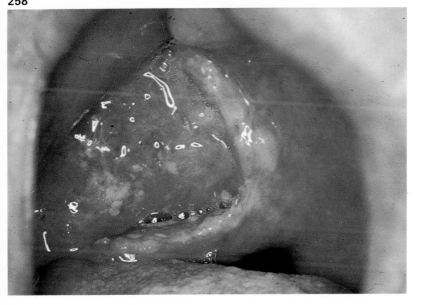

Pharynx

259 Polyp of pharynx The reddish polypi arise high up in the pharynx and are similar to the nasal polypi. They have a stalk and are soft and rubbery in consistency.

260 Pharyngeal pouch This is found in the elderly and may present with dysphagia, regurgitation after meals, or intermittent swelling in the neck. The large pouch is seen coming from the back round the left side of the pharynx.

261 Pharyngeal pouch Typical x-ray after a barium swallow showing the fluid level in the pouch.

259

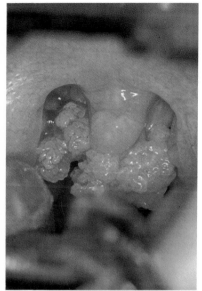

260

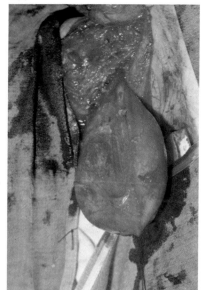

261

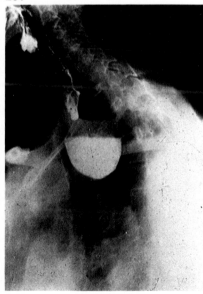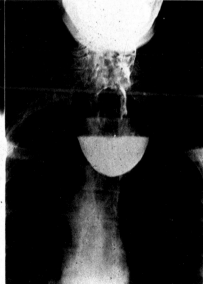

HYPOPHARYNX

Carcinoma of this area is of four types depending on the site; epilaryngeal, piriform fossa, lateral wall, and post-cricoid..

262 Cancer of the piriform fossa This usually presents at a late stage, often as a secondary in the neck. This pharyngogram shows the space-filling lesion.

263 Post-cricoid carcinoma This resected specimen shows the retro-cricoid cancer at the upper end of oesophagus. Usual history is of dysphagia. A barium swallow and direct examination are helpful in diagnosis. They respond to radiotherapy but this one recurred and had to be excised.

263

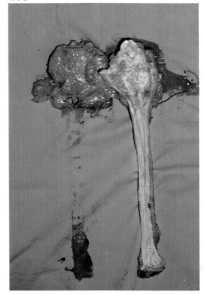

262

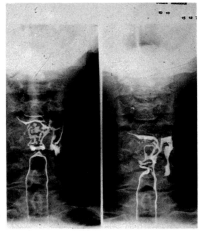

Larynx

264 A laryngocoele is a lateral air containing swelling which is increased by blowing the nose and is easily emptied by pressure.

264

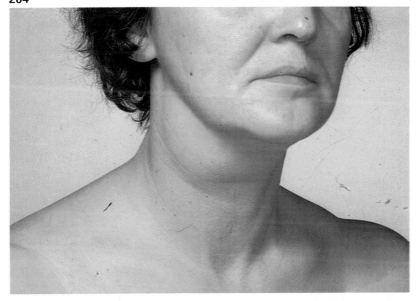

265 Laryngeal polyp appearing as a pearly nodule. The lesion is commonly seen in singers who complain of a tired or husky voice.

266 Carcinoma of larynx produces a huskiness of the voice and enlarged cervical glands. Direct laryngoscopy and biopsy will make the diagnosis. A laryngectomy has been performed with removal of involved glands.

265

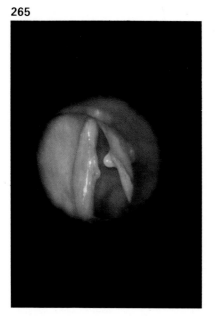

266

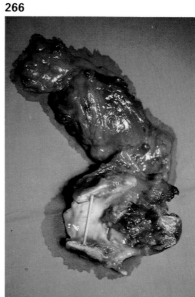

Lesions in the Neck

The surgical conditions of the neck may be classified in a number of different ways. Most of the lesions present as swellings:

CYSTIC SWELLINGS   cystic hygroma, thyroglossal cyst, branchial cyst, sebaceous cyst, pneumatocoele, dermoid cyst.

SOLID SWELLINGS   branchial carcinoma, anaplastic carcinoma, carotid body tumour, lymphoma, lymphatic leukaemia, Hodgkin's disease, secondary cancer, Wryneck, cervical rib.

SWELLINGS OF THYROID

SWELLINGS OF PAROTID

INFLAMMATORY LESIONS

Acute   acute infection submandibular gland, abscess of neck, Ludwig's angina, carbuncle, furuncle, anthrax.

Chronic   tuberculosis abscess, tuberculous glands, syphilis in secondary glands, actinomycosis of neck.

PULSATILE SWELLINGS   aneurysm.

Cystic swellings

267 Cystic hygroma This congenital lymphatic cyst is unilocular or multi-ocular, filled by clear fluid. The swellings are part solid and part cystic. It is prone to attacks of inflammation, and can disappear after a few months. This lesion disappeared without treatment after nine months.

268 Thyroglossal cyst in the middle line of the neck and attached to the hyoid bone or back of tongue.

269 Thyroglossal cyst On protruding the tongue the cyst moves up.

270 Thyroglossal cyst excised. The cyst contains a clear fluid. The upward extension must be carefully excised.

267

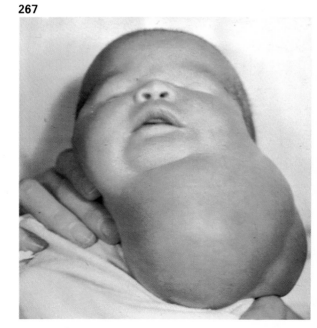

268

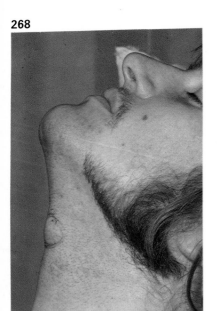

269

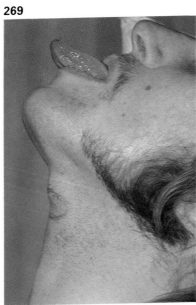

270

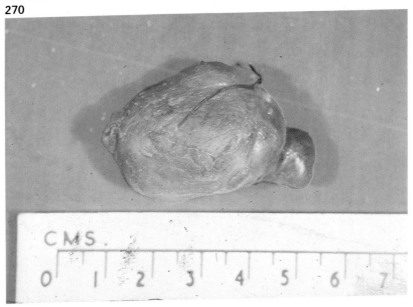

271 Branchial cyst is on one side of the neck commonly in upper part and deep to sternomastoid muscle. It has a clear outline of moderate tension and grows very slowly.

272 Branchial cyst fluid showing the characteristic cholesterol crystals.

273 Sebaceous cyst in midline of neck. The cyst is attached to the skin.

274 Sublingual dermoid cyst is seen in the midline. It occurs in young people and it is not attached to the skin.

275 A pneumatocoele is a rare swelling in the lower part of the anterior triangle of neck. It is soft, elastic, crepitant, and resonant to percussion. The picture on the right shows the swelling distended by coughing which accentuates the herniation of the lung.

271

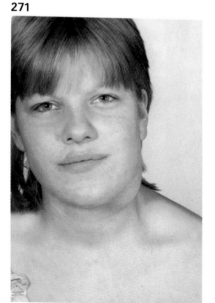

272

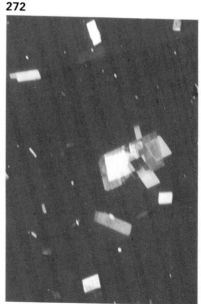

273

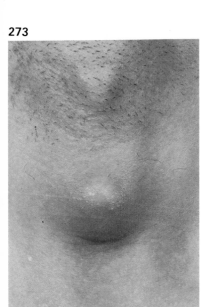

274

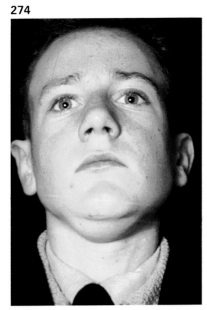

275

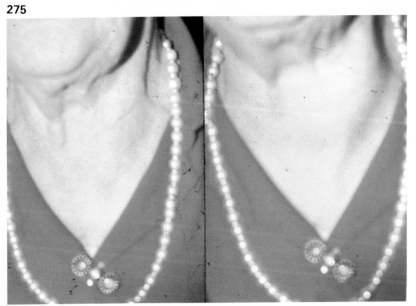

Solid swellings

276 A branchial carcinoma This is a tumour which is very difficult to diagnose. Biopsy is necessary and other conditions must be excluded.

277 Anaplastic carcinoma This began as a solid mass in one side of the neck which grew rapidly to this large size. Biopsy confirmed the lesion. No primary site was found.

278 Anaplastic carcinoma following radiotherapy showing disappearance of the tumour.

279 Hodgkin's disease involving the lymphatic glands in the neck. This is one type of lymphoma where the glands enlarge in groups of quite large size of rubbery consistency without a tendency to infiltrate or suppurate. A periodic moderate type of fever may be present.

280 Lymphatic leukaemia is associated with large masses of glands. The blood picture will confirm the diagnosis.

276

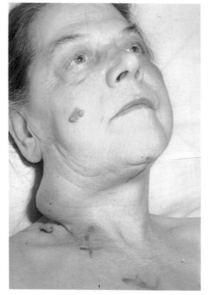

277

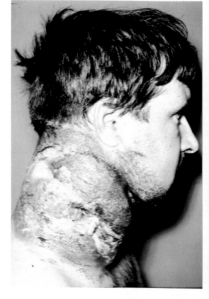

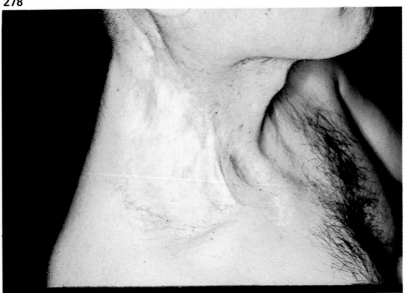

278

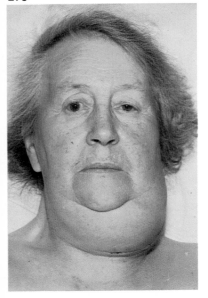

279

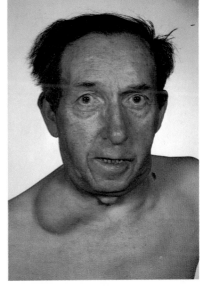

280

281 Squamous cell carcinoma This mass grew and infiltrated rapidly. Biopsy confirmed the diagnosis. No primary site could be found.

282 Wryneck This man had in infancy a mass in the right sternomastoid muscle. The muscle becomes fibrotic. Facial asymmetry may be present.

283 Carotid body tumour These tumours arise from chemoreceptor tissue and are thus chemodactomas. The tumour appears at the level of the carotid bifurcation in the neck. They can be moved from side to side but not up and down. Arteriography shows a widening of space between the internal and external carotid arteries and evidence of a vascular tumour.

284 Cervical rib This sometimes presents as a lump in the posterior triangle of the neck. This patient had a cervical rib on the right side. A slight swelling is present. Diagnosis is confirmed by plain x-ray.

281

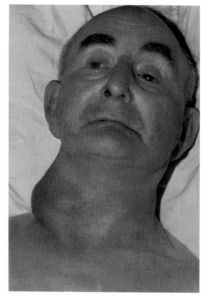

282

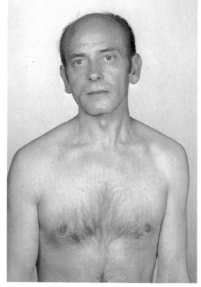

283

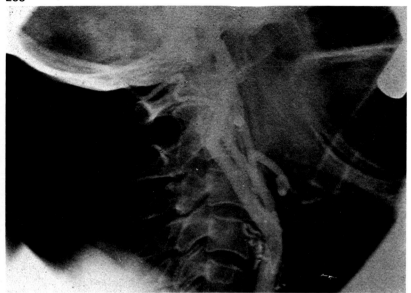

284

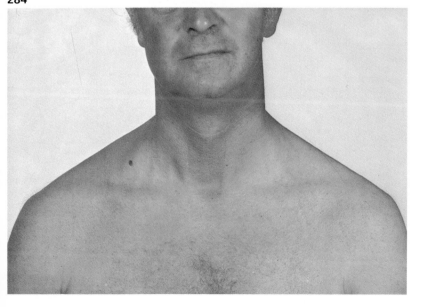

159

Inflammatory lesions

285 Syphilis The glands in the right side of the neck are secondary to a primary chancre in the right side of the lower lip. The chancre cleared up just before the glands appeared.

286 Actinomycosis This curious lesion was thought to be an infected thyroglossal cyst although placed a little low. The pus confirmed the diagnosis.

287 Tuberculous glands are less commonly seen now. They appear as rubbery matted enlarged glands. When they go on to abscess formation the solid mass becomes softer and cystic, and of low tension. The surface becomes reddened, but not oedematous.

Pulsatile swellings

288 Aneurysm In this patient the aneurysm arose in the subclavian artery as a pulsatile swelling above the clavicle. Expansile pulsation was present.

285

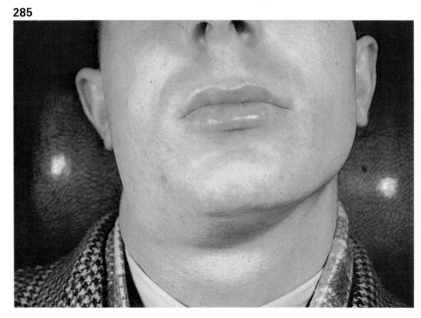

286

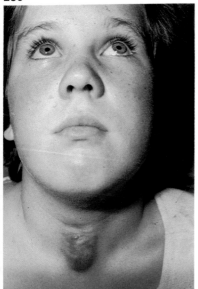

287

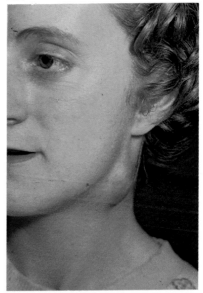

288

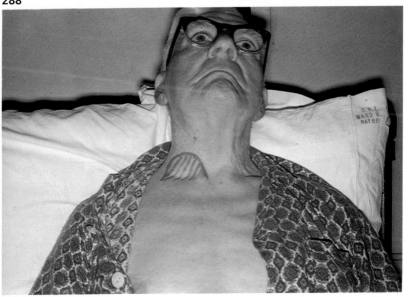

Disease of the Oesophagus

289 Congenital oesophageal atresia This is commonly associated with tracheo-oesophageal fistula. The baby regurgitates his feeds and saliva. The radio-opaque material has stopped in the upper oesophagus; some spill-over may occur into the trachea. The lower oesophagus is connected to the trachea in over 80% of cases so that air passes down to distend the stomach. A catheter passed through the mouth will quickly be arrested in the upper oesophagus.

290 Foreign bodies of various types can be swallowed. Coins and pins and dentures seem to stick easily. The safety pin is illustrated by plain x-ray. Barium swallow may at times be necessary and finally oesophagoscopy. Pain and dysphagia are commonest complaints.

291 Foreign body Even a white horse may be swallowed by children. The second radiograph shows it trotting on although unsure of its way.

289

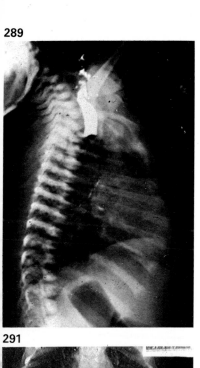

290

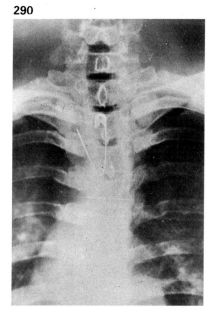

291

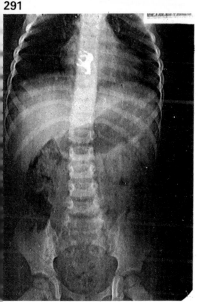

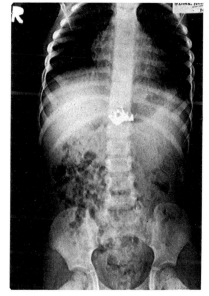

292 Sliding hiatus hernia The clinical features are those of reflux oesophagitis, i.e. burning retrosternal pain (heart-burn), dysphagia, anaemia. The heart-burn is worse on lying or bending down. Barium swallow and oesophagoscopy are diagnostic.

293 Sliding hiatus hernia Line drawing to show the peritoneum covering the gastric protrusion above the diaphragm. This type accounts for over 90% of hiatus hernias.

294 Sliding hiatus hernia At operation the oesophagus can be seen passing through a wide oesophageal hiatus.

295 Sliding hiatus hernia showing the complication of narrowing due to spasm or stricture and a peptic ulcer.

296 Sliding hiatus hernia Line drawing of **295**.

292

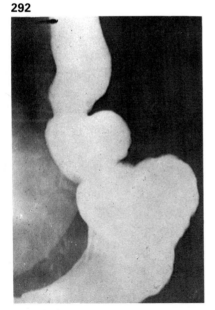

293

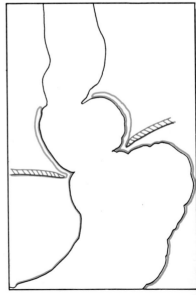

294

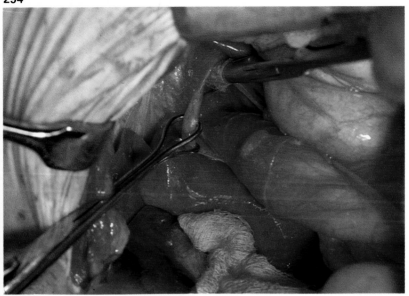

295

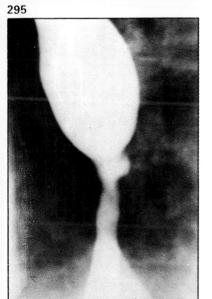

296

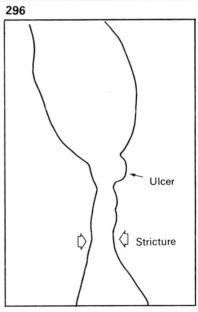

297 Sliding hiatus hernia The narrowed area in the oesophagus is apparent above the gastric extension above the diaphragm. It is a stricture.

298 Sliding hiatus hernia Line drawing of **297**.

299 In paraoesophageal hernia the greater curvature of the stomach has rolled up alongside the oesophagus into the mediastinum. It produces pressure symptoms, intermittent dysphagia and sometimes haematemesis.

300 Paraoesophageal hernia Line drawing of **299**. The oesophago-gastric junction lies below the diaphragm. No reflux oesophagitis.

301 Mixed hernia This is a combination of a hiatus hernia and a para-oesophageal hernia. As the gastro-oesophageal sphincteric mechanism is upset reflux oesophagitis with heartburn will occur.

302 Mixed hernia Line drawing of **301**. The gastro-oesophageal junction is above the diaphragm.

297

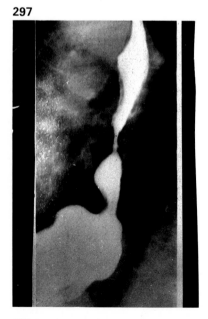

298

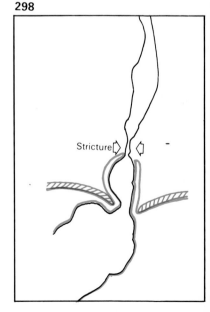

Stricture

299

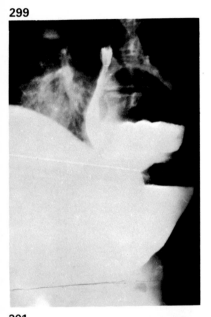

300

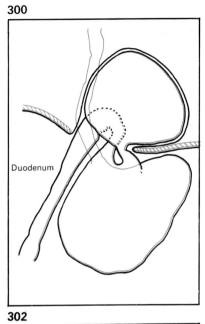

Duodenum

301

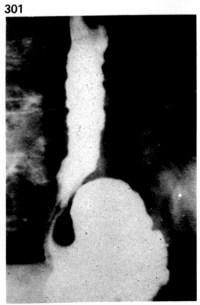

302

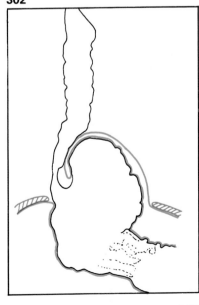

167

303 Achalasia of the oesophagus is commoner in women of middle-age. Dysphagia is the main symptom. Diagnosis is made by barium swallow which shows the dilated oesophagus ending in a conically narrowed, cardio-oesophageal junction. Manometry is sometimes helpful.

304 Achalasia of oesophagus Line drawing of **303** shows the dilated oesophagus ending at the level of the diaphragm.

305 Oesophageal varices The dilated veins in the lower end of the oesophagus are evident. The patient had cirrhosis of the liver with portal hypertension.

306 Oesophageal varices A barium swallow shows the characteristic appearance of dilated oesophageal veins.

303

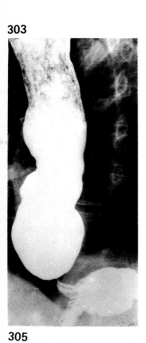

304

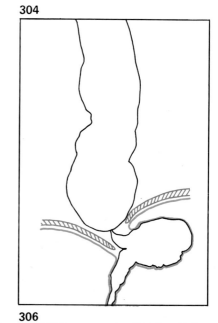

305

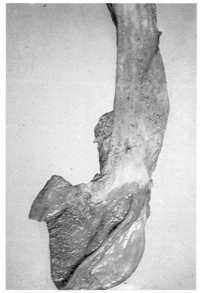

306

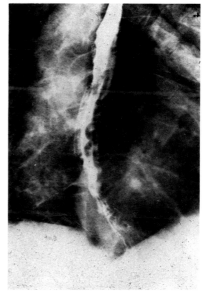

307 Leiomyoma of oesophagus is the commonest of the rare benign tumours of the oesophagus. A mild dysphagia is common. Barium swallow and oesophagoscopy confirm the diagnosis. This is a resected specimen.

308 Carcinoma of lower oesophagus produces a progressive dysphagia of solids to liquids with weight loss. The barium swallow shows the typical picture of narrowing with a shelf-like upper border.

307

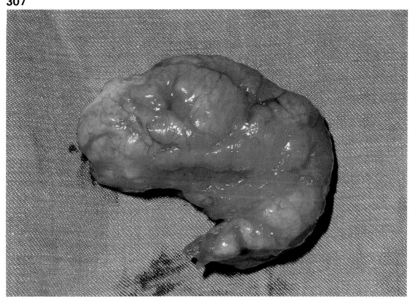

308

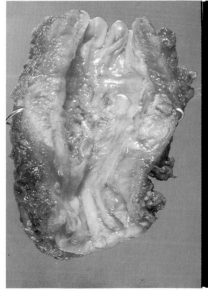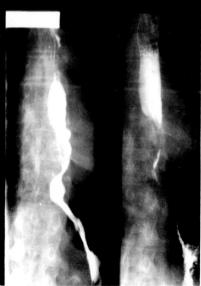

Abdominal Pain and Lesions of the Stomach

Pain is the commonest symptom that brings a patient to the surgeon. Analysis of abdominal pain may therefore help considerably in diagnosis. We begin by asking the following questions:

- *Where did the pain start?*

- *Where is it now?*

- *What type of pain is it (dull ache, colic, excruciating)?*

- *How long has it been present?*

- *Is it continuous or does it vary?*

- *Does anything relieve it or make it worse?*

- *Is it associated with nausea or vomiting or with a desire to micturate or defaecate?*

- *Is it associated with shock?*

The alimentary canal developed from a single tube down the midline of the body and the pain pathways were laid down before the tube elongated and developed its offshoots. True visceral pain of alimentary origin is therefore felt in the midline as seen in **309**.

When the inflammation extends through the organ to involve the peritoneum or the surroundings the pain experienced is now somatic pain, and is felt at the site of the organ which is also the area of maximum tenderness. This is the so-called shift of pain.

Stomach and duodenal pain starts in the epigastrium and the tenderness is also there over the ulcer. Appendicular pain, by contrast, starts in the area of the middle third of the linea alba, but when extension involves the peritoneum the pain 'shifts' to the site of the organ.

The student may be caught out by small bowel pain due to an incarcerated femoral hernia. The pain is felt in the area of the middle third of the linea alba, while on examination the tender area is a small swelling in the femoral triangle. Large bowel pain is felt vaguely across the lower abdomen and in the left iliac fossa in the case of diverticutitis. Gallbladder pain is felt first in the epigastrium but shifts to the right hypochondrium and passes through to the back.

Back pain may indicate the acute abdomen (**310**). A penetrating duodenal ulcer passes through to the back on the right, but lower down than gallbladder pain. Acute pancreatitis may give rise to severe back pain passing to the left, as may a ruptured aortic aneurysm at an even lower site. A slipped disc may on rare occasions be diagnosed in error for a ruptured aneurysm as the areas of pain may merge.

309 Visceral pain is felt in the midline as the gut originates as a midline structure, and as far as the brain is concerned remains so.

309

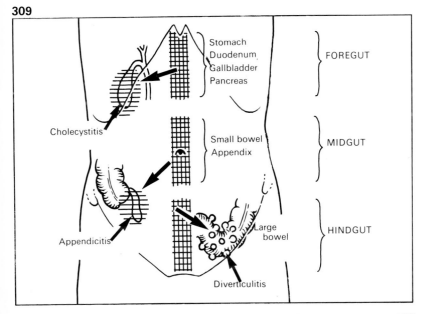

310 Back pain is due to the disease process involving nerves in the retroperitoneal area.

311 Hypertrophic pyloric stenosis The thickening of the pyloric muscle occurs usually in males and the symptoms of projectile non-bilious vomiting appear at about two to four weeks of age. The gastric distension is shown here.

310

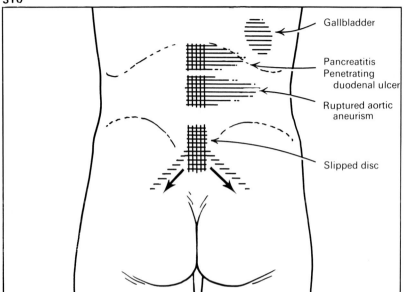

Gallbladder

Pancreatitis
Penetrating
  duodenal ulcer

Ruptured aortic
aneurism

Slipped disc

311

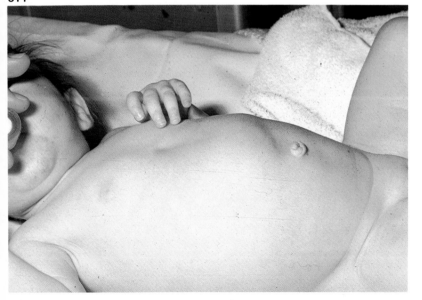

312 Hypertrophic pyloric stenosis With feeding a wave of peristalsis may be seen passing across the epigastrium and the 'tumour' of the pylorus may be felt.

313 Gastric ulcer The stomach is opened along the greater curvature to show the ulceration on the lesser curvature. Symptoms of epigastric pain half an hour after meals led to a barium meal and gastroscopy which clinched the diagnosis.

312

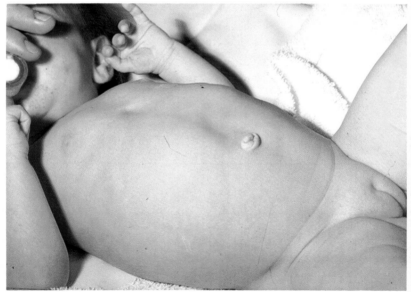

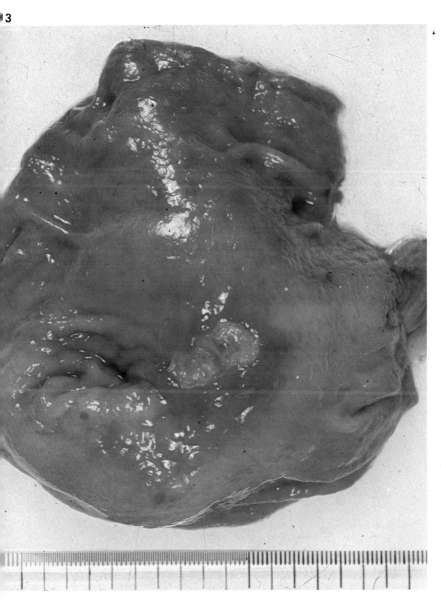

314 Gastric ulcer This is clearly shown as a constant area in a number of films where the barium has been localised. Gastroscopy also confirmed the presence of an ulcer at this site.

315 Gastric ulcer: haematemesis This ulcer illustrates the characteristic features of a benign ulcer. In one part is a dark spot. This is the clot in the vessel which bled so much that partial gastrectomy was required.

316 Gastric ulcer: hourglass stomach This large chronic gastric ulcer has produced a contraction of the middle of the stomach with an hourglass type deformity. It is most often seen in women and in association with pyloric stenosis.

317 Hourglass stomach The barium meal shows the typical constriction.

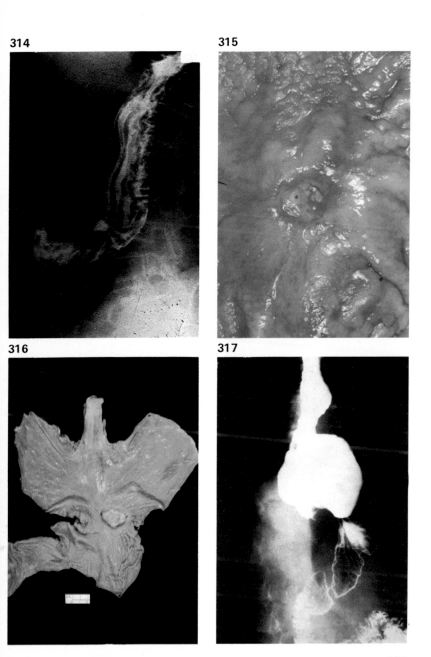

318 Pyloric stenosis Dilatation of the stomach may be congenital as mentioned or due to a duodenal ulcer or gastric carcinoma. This patient vomited undigested food in large amounts. A stricture from a duodenal ulcer was found at operation.

318

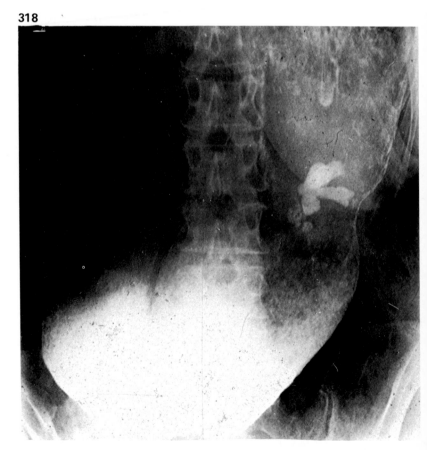

319 Gastric ulcer: malignant change Controversy exists as to whether gastric ulcers may on rare cases become malignant, or small carcinomas undergo ulceration due to acid pepsin digestion with evidence of healing on treatment. In this patient what looked like an ordinary chronic ulcer was confirmed by histology as malignant.

319

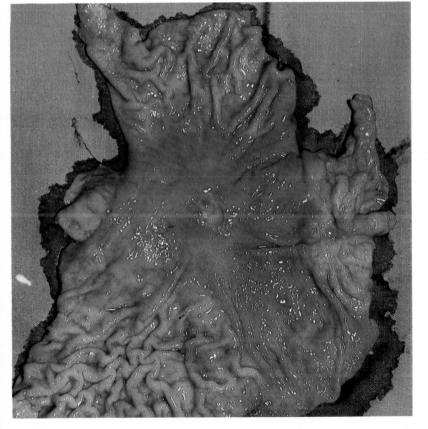

320 A hair ball occurs rarely when hair is swallowed by the patient and accumulates in the stomach. The distension on the left side of the epigastrium is the notable feature.

321 A hair ball A barium meal outlining the hair ball.

322 A hair ball removed from the stomach of the case in **321**. Neoplasms of the stomach are the benign polyp (single or multiple) which must be distinguished from the polypoid carcinoma, and the leiomyoma. The malignant tumours are nearly always the carcinoma, but sometimes a lymphoma or leiomyosarcoma may be present.

323 Polyposis of stomach This patient presented with anaemia due to blood loss. The diagnosis was suggested by the barium meal appearances and confirmed at operation. No malignancy was present.

320

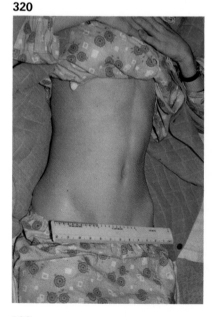

321

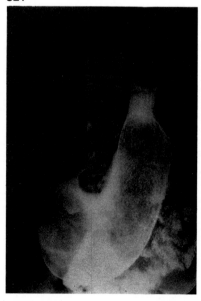

322

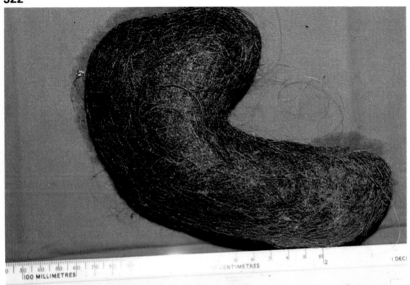

323

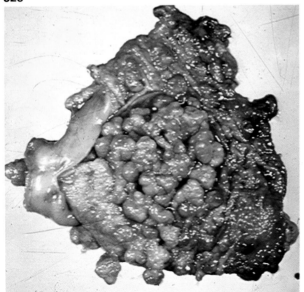

324 Cancer of stomach This cancer was found in a patient who had a vague dyspepsia, anorexia and loss of weight. A mass was felt in the epigastrium as it may be in about 20–25% of cases. Diagnosis was confirmed by barium meal and gastroscopy.

325 Troisier's node in cancer of the stomach. This is a metastasis in the supraclavicular gland due to spread along the thoracic duct. It is a very late sign and is rarely felt.

326 A leiomyosarcoma of stomach These usually arise in midpart of the stomach and often grow to a large size. The mass may be felt on examination especially if it grows outwards into the abdominal cavity. If it grows into the gastric lumen a barium meal will be useful.

324

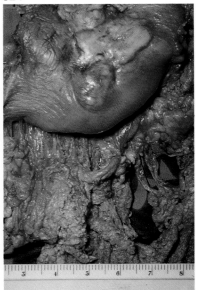

325

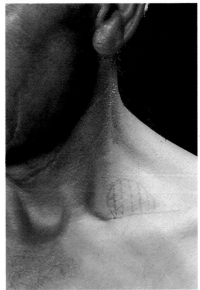

326

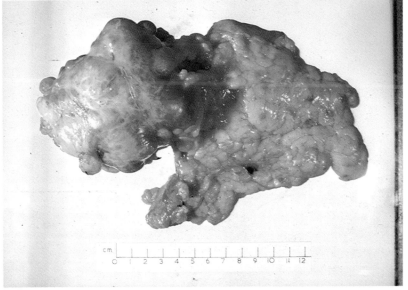

327 Volvulus of the stomach is rare. This patient had sudden attacks of epigastric pain and vomiting. In two attacks he was thought to have coronary thrombosis. On the third attack a barium meal made the diagnosis showing the obvious displacement of the stomach.

328 A stomach ulcer appears months to years after a gastro-jejunal anastomosis. The recurrent pain is like the previous ulcer but often more severe and is felt on the left side of the epigastrium. Vomiting is common. Barium meal is helpful but can miss the lesion. Gastroscopy should clinch the diagnosis.

327

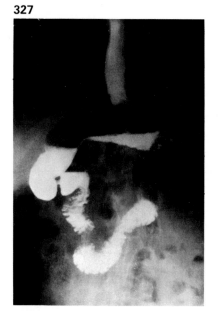

328

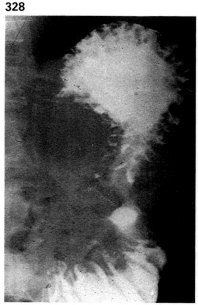

Disease of the Duodenum

329 Congenital duodenal obstruction presented in this infant with bilious vomiting shortly after birth. Distension of the abdomen was most marked in epigastrium. Diagnosis was made by x-ray and confirmed at operation.

330 Duodenal ulcer A small ulcer is shown in the resected specimen. It produced epigastrium pain two to three hours after meals relieved by food and alkalies. Epigastric tenderness was noted. Gastric acid secretion was raised. Diagnosis was confirmed by barium meal and duodenoscopy.

329

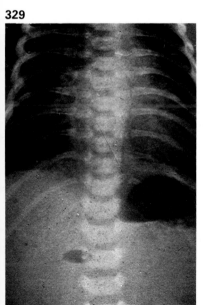

330

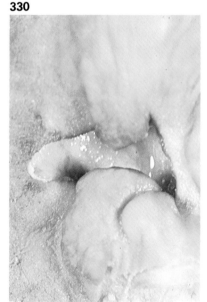

331 Congenital duodenal obstruction The plain x-ray showed an air bubble in the stomach and another in the duodenal area – the double-bubble sign. The presence of gas lower down in the intestine suggested that the obstruction was incomplete – a stenosis rather than an atresia.

332 Pyloric stenosis is a complication of duodenal ulcer in which vomiting of undigested food is a feature. Bile is absent from the vomit. Dehydration, weight loss, and metabolic alkalosis may be present to a varying degree. On examination a succussion splash can be elicited and a barium meal presents a typical picture of retention of barium in the stomach which in this case was enormous. An incidental stag horn calculus is visible.

333 Carcinoma of the duodenum is rare. The most common site is in the region of the ampulla of Vater as shown in the specimen of a pancreaticoduodenectomy. A vague upper abdominal pain may be present but the characteristic features are intermittent jaundice, anaemia, and occult blood in the stool. A barium meal is helpful in that it may show a reversed figure three appearance.

331

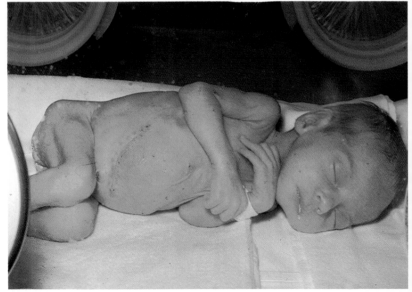

332

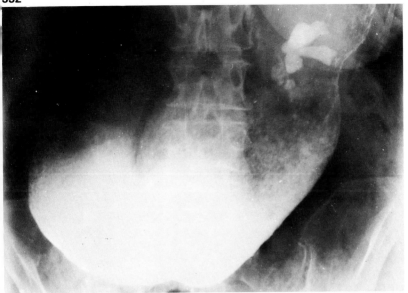

333

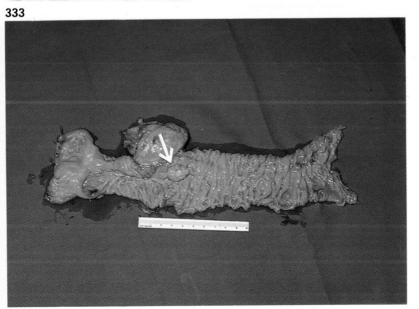

334 Cancer of the duodenum may occur elsewhere as in the supra-ampullary portion. The ampulla is denoted by the stick. Pain, anaemia, and an abdominal mass may be more prominent than with ampullary cancer. If large, obstructive jaundice may be present. A duodenoscopy or a barium meal will establish the diagnosis.

334

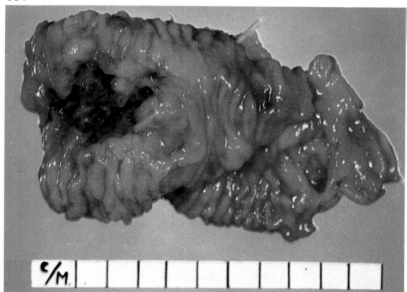

Lesions of the Small Bowel

335 Congenital obstruction of ileum The baby vomited green bile, had abdominal distension and passed no meconium. Intestinal patterning was visible and could be felt by the 'feather touch'. Confirmation of diagnosis was made by plain x-ray of abdomen which gives some idea of the level of obstruction.

336 Congenital obstruction of ileum The distension of much of the small bowel is evident as is the abnormally narrow colon on barium enema.

335

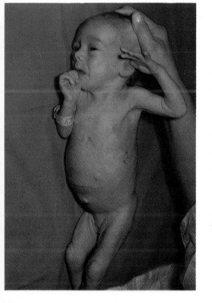

336

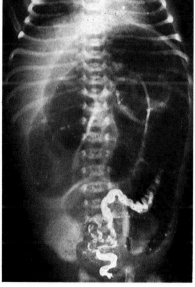

337 Volvulus neonatorum presents with bilious vomiting, pain and very marked abdominal distension. The gross distension of the jejunum is obvious with the collapsed bowel below. The bowel also shows well the valvular conniventes which are seen on x-ray and denote distended jejunum.

338 Meconium ileus The infant had a distended abdomen, vomited bile, and passed no meconium. The abdomen appeared shiny and reddened. Plain x-ray showed distended loops of bowel and a soap-bubble appearance due to admixture of air and meconium. The enlarged bowel full of viscid meconium is apparent.

339 Vitello-intestinal duct may open at the umbilicus discharging small bowel contents. An injection into the fistula of contrast material will establish the diagnosis.

340 A Meckel's diverticulum is usually found at operation for appendicitis. It is present in about two per cent of the population and may give rise to no problems but complications can occur.

337

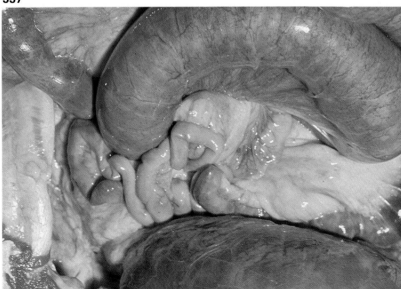

338

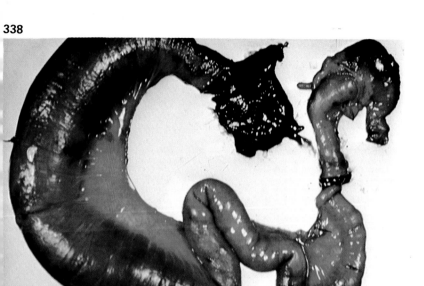

339

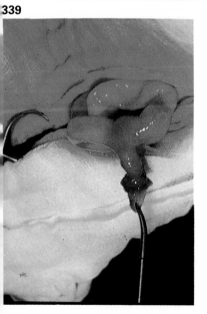

340

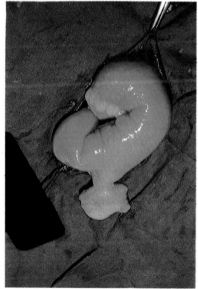

341 Meckel's diverticulitis As in the appendix, inflammation may occur. The signs and symptoms are identical to acute appendicitis. The tenderness may be more medial.

342 Meckel's diverticulitis This shows gross enlargement of the end of the diverticulum. Gangrene and perforation may occur. A palpable mass was present.

343 A Meckel's diverticulum may be filled by orange pith and produce obstruction. The dilater proximal bowel is evident. Diagnosis is made at operation.

341

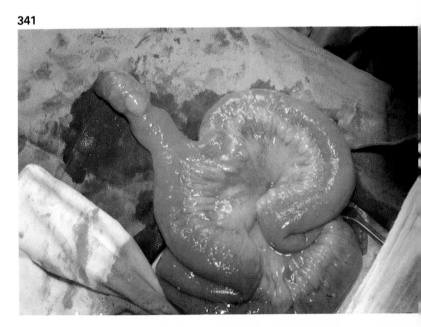

342

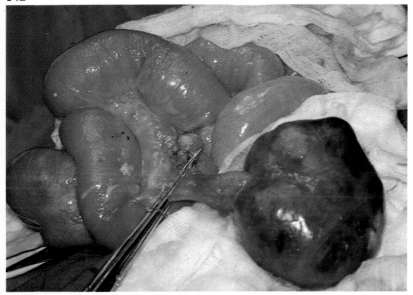

343

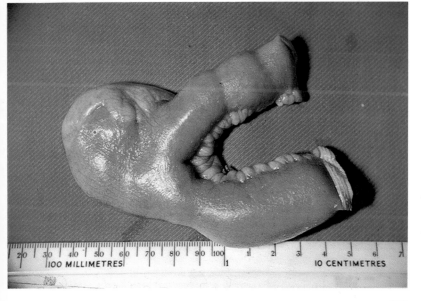

344 Meckel's diverticulum may contain aberrant gastric mucosa which may be strong enough to produce ulceration at the junction with the ileum. Pain after meals and tenderness in right iliac fossa may be present and occult blood may be found in the faeces.

345 Meckel's diverticulum with acute ulcer This may bleed or perforate and is difficult to diagnose before operation.

346 Jejunal diverticula are present in the mesenteric border. They may be symptomless but may become inflamed with complications, or may become filled with food and cause an obstruction.

344

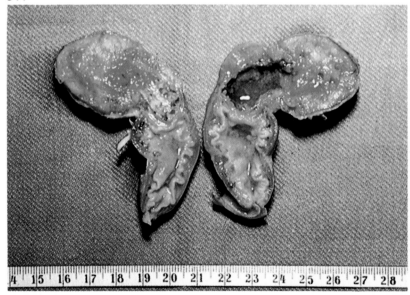

345

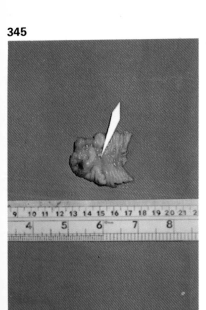

346

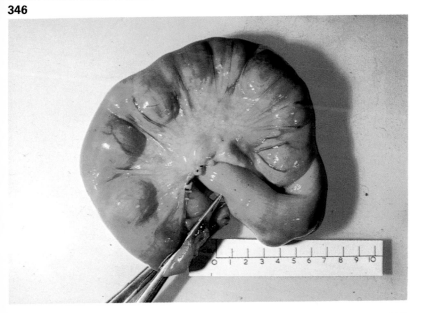

347 Jejunal diverticulitis This resected specimen shows the inflamed diverticula. Patient had central periumbilical pain and marked tenderness round the umbilicus. Unless patient is known to have diverticula or they are shown on barium meal, it is difficult to diagnose before operation.

348 Acute appendicitis usually presents with central, peri-umbilical pain and tenderness in the right iliac fossa. Later pain is also experienced at the site of tenderness due to extension of the inflammation to the parietal peritoneum.

349 Appendicitis may result from obstruction of the appendix by a faecolith. Distal appendix is going gangrenous. Pain and tenderness will be most marked in the right iliac fossa.

347

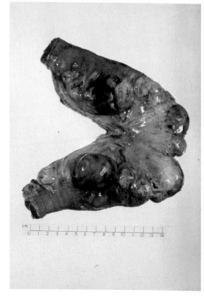

348

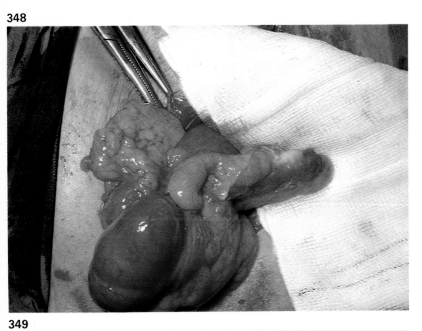

349

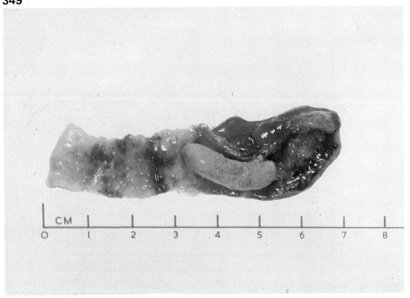

350 Appendix abscess The symptoms of appendicitis are followed by a pyrexia, sweats, a tender mass in the right iliac fossa and a leucocytosis. The mass is outlined.

351 Shingles may lead to misdiagnosis of appendicitis. Patient may complain of severe pain in right loin and right iliac fossa. The pain may precede the appearance of the typical skin lesion.

352 Enteritis necroticans is a severe infection of the small bowel due to a *Welchii* organism. The patient, in whom the resected specimen was removed, had severe abdominal pain, toxaemia, and collapse. Diagnosis made at operation.

350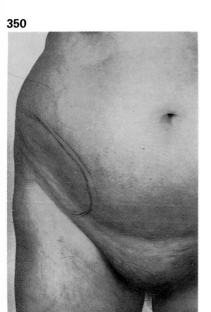

351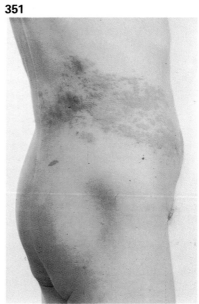

352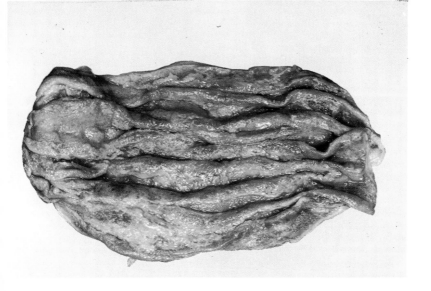

353 Pseudomembranous enterocolitis affects small and large bowel due sometimes to overgrowth of staphylococci as a result of antibiotic therapy. Diarrhoea, abdominal pain, and toxaemia were present in this case.

354 Crohn's disease is a chronic inflammatory disorder of the alimentary tract. It usually affects the ileum less commonly the colon. The wall of the bowel and the mesentery are thickened. The granulomatous change in the bowel is seen in this specimen.

355 Crohn's disease may present like an acute appendicitis or may be characterised by diarrhoea, abdominal pain, low grade fever, anaemia, weight loss and a palpable mass. Diagnosis is confirmed by a small bowel enema.

353

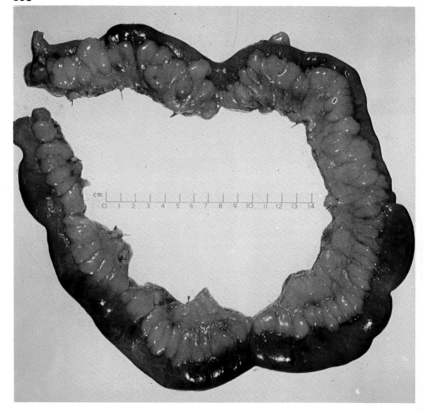

354

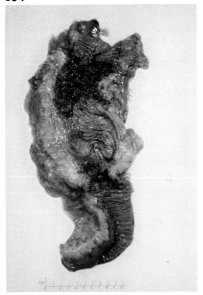

355

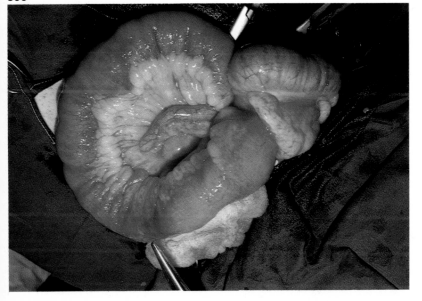

356 Crohn's disease This pathological specimen shows the characteristic thickening of the wall and narrowing of the lumen. On the left is the thickened narrow terminal ileum which gives rise to Stierlin's sign on barium enema.

357 Tuberculosis of ileum is not common in western countries. It may appear like Crohn's disease as a granulomatous condition or in an ulcerative form. This patient had diarrhoea and acute abdominal pain.

358 Ileal tuberculosis The caseating glands in the mesentery support the diagnosis in patient in **357**. Tubercle bacilli were found in the glands and resected specimen.

356

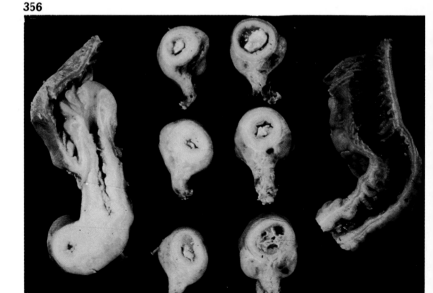

357

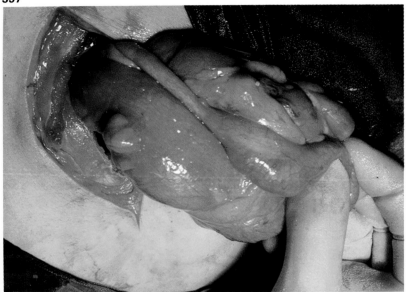

358

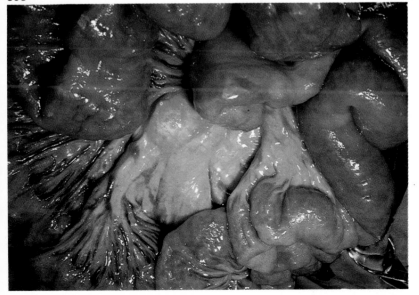

359 Mesenteric adenitis This condition of inflammatory enlargement of the lymphatic glands due to coccobacilli of *Yersinia* group. It occurs usually in children who have recurrent abdominal pain and tenderness in periumbilical region and R.I.F. When the patient turns onto the left side the tenderness shifts to the left indicating that the mesenteric glands are involved and differentiating the condition from acute appendicitis.

360 Acute mesenteric vascular occlusion may be due to obstruction of artery or vein. It gives rise to severe diffuse abdominal pain, nausea, vomiting and sometimes a bloody diarrhoea. Slight tenderness was present in this case to begin with but increased later. Toxaemia and circulatory collapse occurred.

361 Small bowel obstruction illustrating the typical ladder pattern which occurs in lower small bowel obstruction. In jejunal obstruction bilious vomiting is dominant and the ladder pattern absent.

362 Post-appendicectomy obstruction There are many causes of small bowel obstruction. One of the commonest is adhesions following a previous appendicectomy. The clinical features are central abdominal pain, vomiting, and abdominal distension and constipation.

359

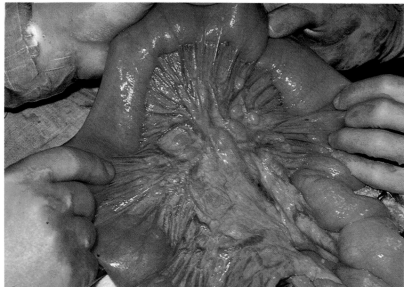

360

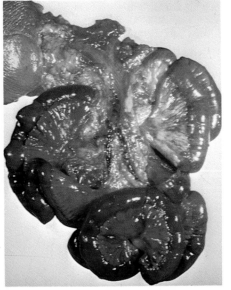

361

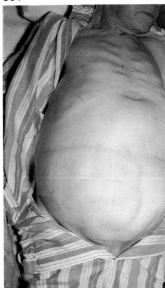

362

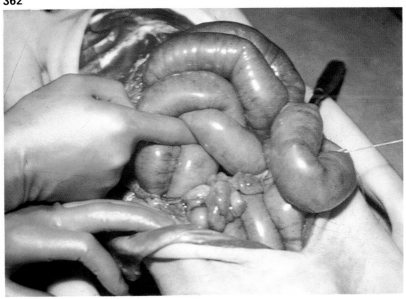

363 Ileo-ileal intussusception due to a benign ileal polyp may produce obstruction. Intussusception is commonest in children at about six months of age who have the clinical features of obstruction and may have a red currant jelly stool.

364 A Richter's hernia in which only part of the wall of the bowel is incorporated in the hernia may produce a partial obstruction and is easily missed. Central abdominal pain, toxaemia and a tender area over a hernial site may be the only clinical features.

365 Gallstone ileus is an uncommon cause of obstruction usually seen in elderly women. The gallstone ulcerated through a cholecyst-duodenal fistula to impact in lower small bowel. A history of gallbladder disease followed by intermittent and finally complete obstruction suggests this as a cause.

366 Enterolith obstruction The enterolith may come from a small gall-stone enlarging in the intestine, or from a duodenal or jejunal diverticulum. The presentation is that of simple obstruction and the diagnosis is made at operation.

363

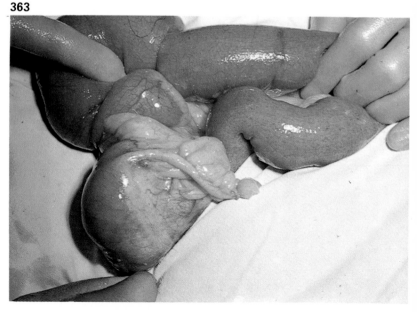

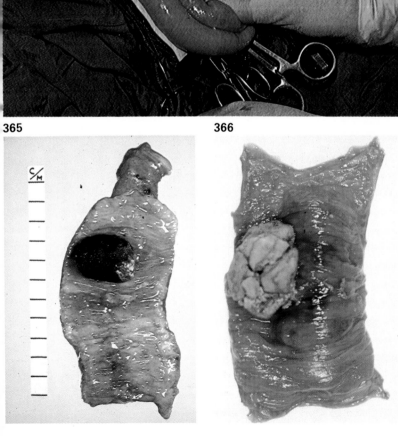

364

365

366

367 Henoch-Schönlein purpura This boy had acute abdominal pain and at operation was found to have a bleeding into the wall of the small bowel. The characteristic rash appeared later. The platelets were normal.

367

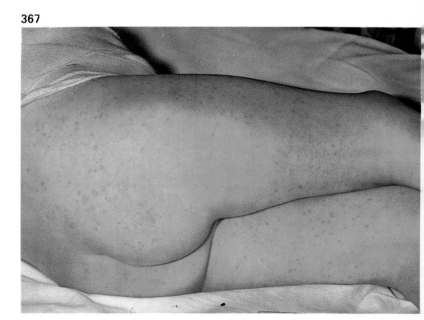

Tumours of small intestine

These are uncommon and form less than five per cent of all tumours of the gastrointestinal tract. The diagnosis of these tumours is difficult. The benign ones are found at operation or may cause obstruction either by their size or forming the apex of an intussusception.

The malignant tumours may also obstruct or perforate or be found on investigation of an obscure anaemia with occult blood in the stool.

Benign	**Malignant**
Single polyp	Adenocarcinoma
Multiple polyps	Lymphosarcoma
Haemangioma	Metastases
Lipoma	Carcinoid
Leiomyoma	

368 Multiple polyposis May appear as part of the Peutz-Jeghers syndrome or Gardener's syndrome. In this patient intestinal bleeding and colicky abdominal pain led to resection. Diagnosis was confirmed by a small bowel enema.

368

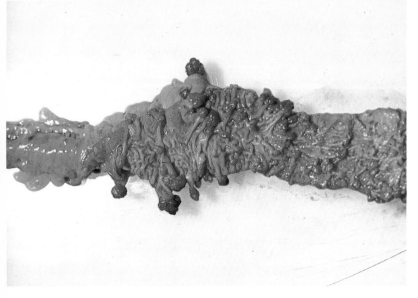

369 Leiomyoma of small bowel may be asymptomatic. This one caused colickly abdominal pain due to obstruction. A tender mass could be felt.

370 Submucosal lipoma This simple tumour was the apex of an intussusception.

371 Carcinoma of small bowel although rare is commoner in the jejunum. In this pathological specimen the tumour had obstructed the ileum and was removed by a right hemicolectomy.

372 Carcinoma of small bowel may present as a perforation with diffuse peritonitis.

369

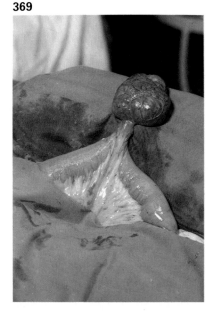

370

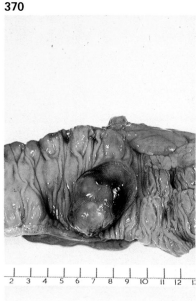

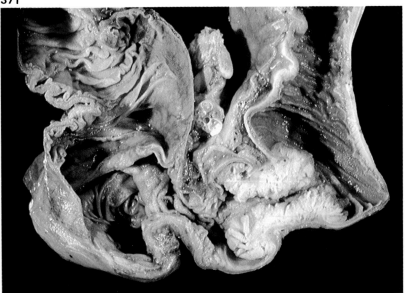

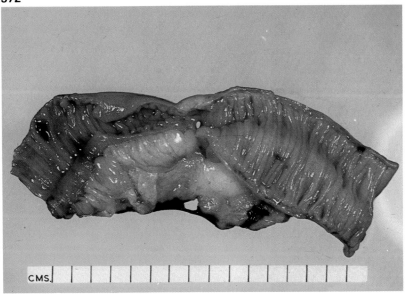

373 Leiomyosarcoma of ileum presented with intestinal obstruction and blood in the stool. A mass was palpable. Diagnosis was made at operation.

374 Primary lymphosarcoma is one of a group of tumours classified as reticulosis. The patient with lesions suffered from abdominal pain, anorexia, loss of weight and anaemia. A large mass was palpable.

375 Lymphosarcoma usually arises in the terminal ileum and as it infiltrates the submucosa may produce a rigid segment. In this case two areas of bowel were affected. The lymph nodes were not grossly enlarged.

376 Carcinoid tumour This is shown in the small bowel where it is regarded as a malignant neoplasm. In the appendix, where it is commoner, it is nearly always benign. This small tumour was the primary. Secondaries were present in the liver and the patient had the carcinoid syndrome.

373

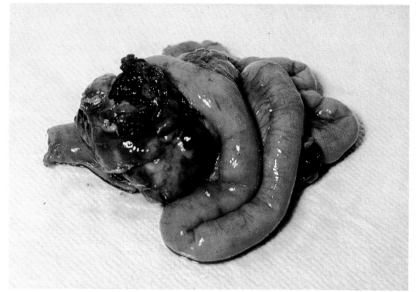

374

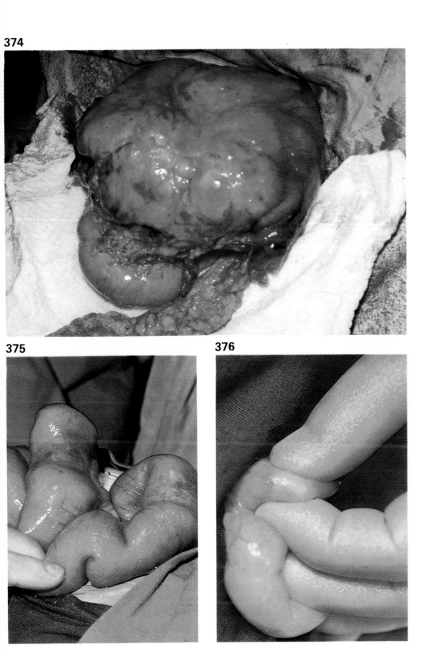

375

376

377 Carcinoid glands removed in the above case. The glands were larger than the primary tumour.

378 Carcinoid in the liver The extensive replacement of the liver was suspected by flushing, diarrhoea, breathless attacks, and a rash in the face which became noticeably redder during attacks.

379 Carcinoid facies The typical malar flush is shown. The urine 5-hydroxyindolacetic acid (5–HIAA) was raised in this patient. Although diagnostic when raised, a normal level does not exclude the condition.

377

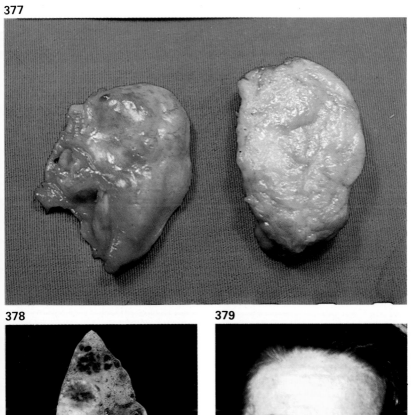

378

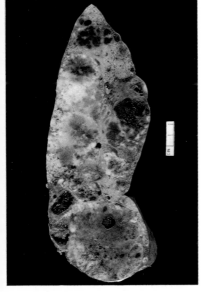

379

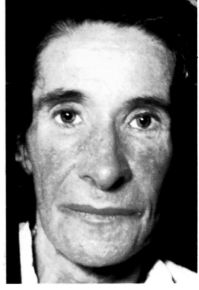

Mesenteric swellings

380 A mesenteric cyst presented as an abdominal swelling without pain. The cystic swelling moved freely in the abdomen especially at right angles to the line of attachment of the mesentery.

381 Torsion of mesenteric cyst and omentum Torsion of omentum is rare but can occur especially in an area containing a cyst. The patient complained of sudden severe abdominal pain and a large tender mass was felt. Intestinal obstruction may be present due to drag on bowel or pressure.

380

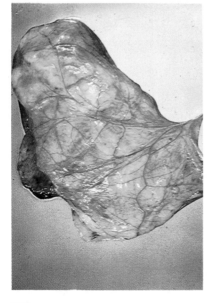

381

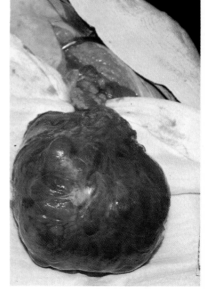

Retroperitoneal lesions

382 A retroperitoneal cyst may arise from remnants of the Wolffian duct or may be teratomatous. They may grow to a very large size as here where the transverse colon is stretched across it. The lesion presented as a cystic abdominal mass and had to be differentiated from a hydronephrosis by an I.V.P.

382

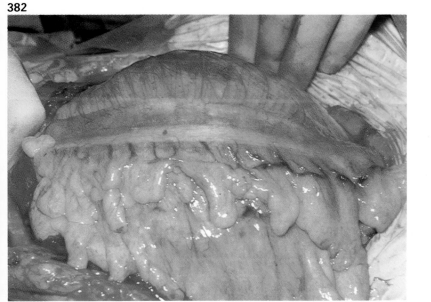

383 Retroperitoneal tumour may be a benign lipoma or a sarcoma. The clinical features are vague abdominal pain and an enlarging mass. In this case the biopsy revealed a seminoma – secondary from a tiny tumour in the left testis which passed unnoticed at general examination. In an obscure abdominal mass examine the testes carefully.

383

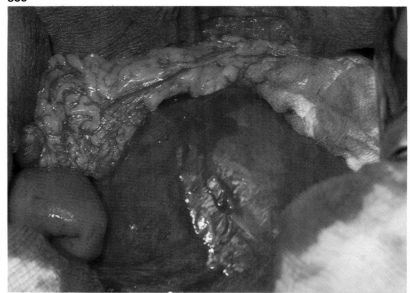

Disease of the Large Bowel

384 Hirschsprung's disease is commoner in males. This little boy passed only a minute amount of meconium within 24 hours of birth. Progressive abdominal distension occurred which was partially relieved by rectal examination.

384

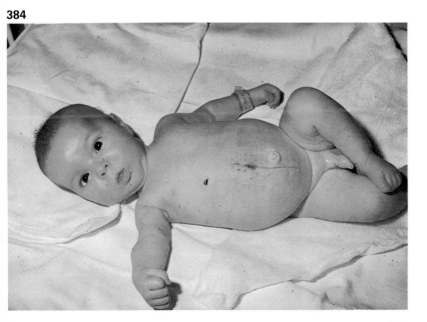

385 Hirschsprung's disease The barium enema demonstrates the narrow aganglionic segment especially in pelvic colon with proximal dilatation. A rectal biopsy confirmed the absence of ganglion cells.

386 Hirschsprung's disease A colostomy was performed early in infancy to relieve the abdominal distension. Definitive operation was done when child was about 10 Kg.

387 Ulcerative colitis is characterised by diarrhoea with passage of blood and mucus. Proctoscopy reveals a reddened granular friable mucosa and barium enema may show lack of haustrations. The granular proctitis is evident in the specimen.

388 Ulcerative colitis The gross hyperaemia shown here results in the bloody diarrhoea so characteristic of the disease. So also is lower abdominal pain, anaemia, loss of weight and fever.

385

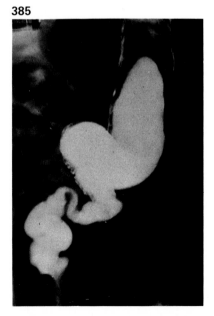

386

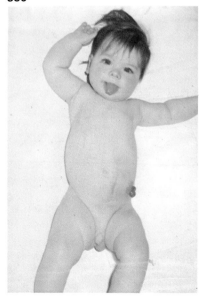

387

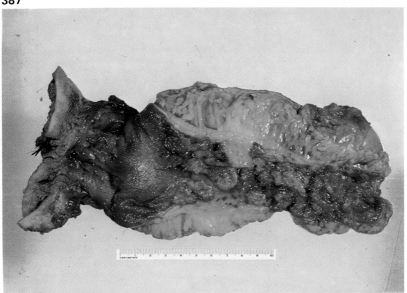

388

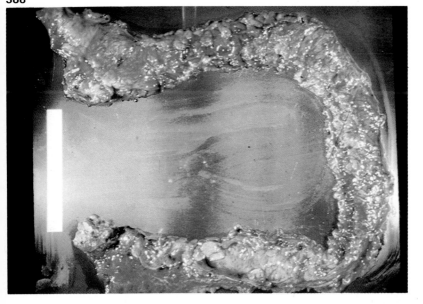

389 Pathological specimen of ulcerative colitis shows very well the loss of mucosa. The intervening areas could appear rather like polyps – the pseudopolyps of ulcerative colitis or produce a characteristic appearance on barium enema.

390 Ulcerative colitis The barium enema shows the characteristic picture of lack of haustrations and irregularity of the edge of the bowel suggesting ulceration.

391 Ulcerative colitis with carcinoma The occurrence of cancer is usually seen in patients who have had the disease for more than 10 years. It is difficult to diagnose clinically but may be shown up in barium enema.

389

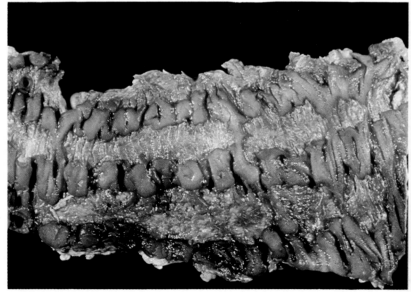

390

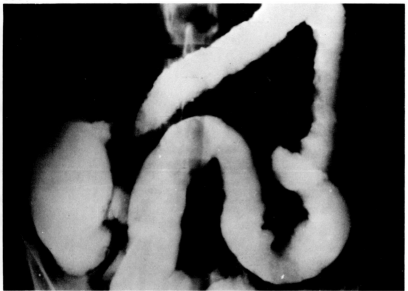

391

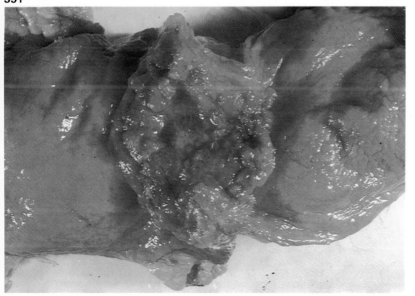

392 Crohn's disease of the colon usually affects only a segment, but skip lesions may be present. The proximal colon is involved in this case. The symptoms are similar to ulcerative colitis with which it may be confused. Barium enema may show the isolated segment involved and a characteristic appearance.

392

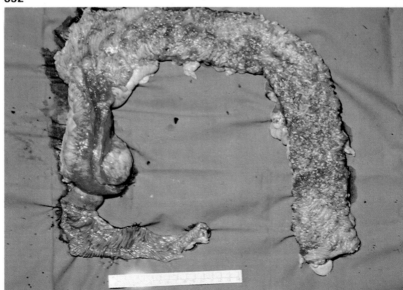

393 Crohn's disease of colon The features on the barium enema are the narrowed areas of the ascending and transverse colon with normal bowel in between.

393

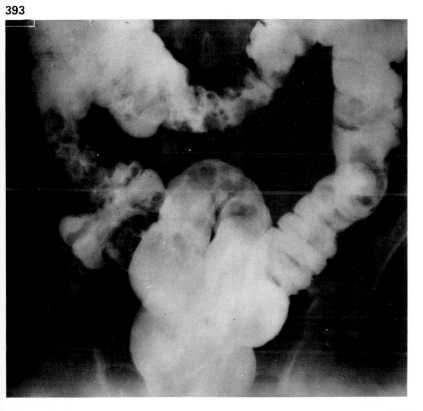

394 Ischaemic colitis may follow resection of an aortic aneurysm where the inferior mesenteric artery is tied off. The patient develops diarrhoea on the third to fifth day after operation. The gangrenous sigmoid colon is shown.

394

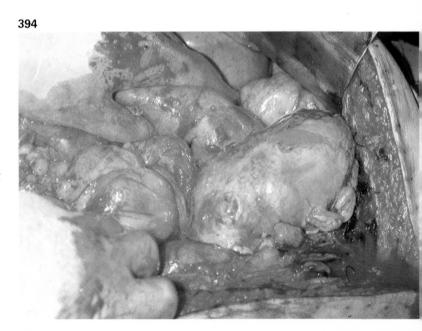

395 Diverticulosis affects mainly the distal colon but may occur throughout. The patient complains of lower abdominal pain and is tender in the left iliac fossa. Constipation is common and sometimes severe haemorrhage occurs.

395

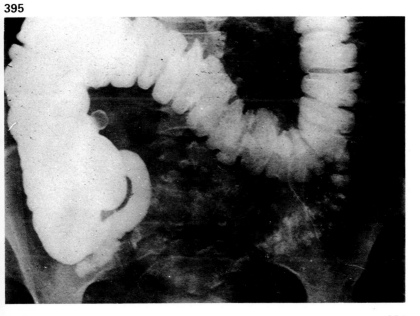

396 Volvulus of colon presents with colicky lower abdominal pain, distension and vomiting in the middle aged to elderly. A plain x-ray shows the characteristic gross distension of the bowel. The exact picture varies with a caecal or sigmoid volvulus. In this case the volvulus involves the sigmoid colon.

396

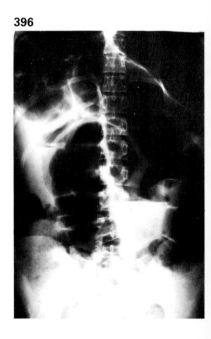

397 Volvulus sigmoid colon A barium enema demonstrates the lower end of the obstruction with the very markedly distended bowel above. No barium could ascend beyond the twist.

397

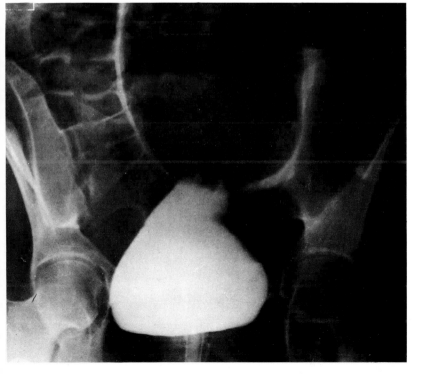

398 Pneumatosis coli presented in this patient with constipation and a feeling of something in the rectum. On P.R. a curious mass was felt all round the rectal wall with smooth nodules. These were seen on sigmoidoscopy to be superficial cysts which burst easily with a loud plop. Barium enema showed an extensive lesion with 'cystic' areas growing, as it were, from the wall of the colon.

398

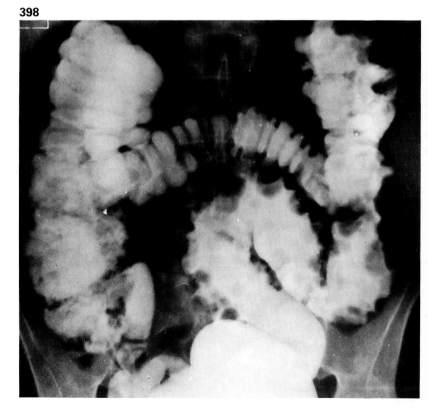

Tumours of large bowel

Benign
Polyp
Lipoma
Leiomyoma
Carcinoid
Various

Malignant
Carcinoma
Lymphosarcoma
Melanoma

BENIGN TUMOURS

These are rare except for the polyp which should strictly be a pedunculated tumour arising from the mucosa. They are usually roughly classified as pedunculated polyps with a long stalk (benign) and the sessile polyp which may be an adenoma or carcinoma.

399 Benign pedunculated polyp of colon may be asymptomatic. In this case the history was of occasional spotting of the faeces with red blood.

399

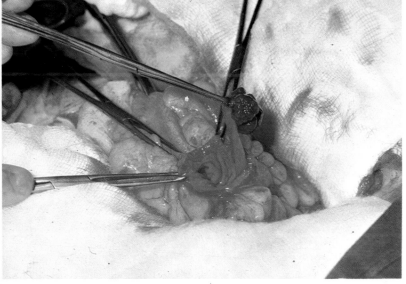

400 A benign polyp is often seen in association with a carcinoma. This raises the controversial question of the polyp being premalignant. Present opinion is negative, although an adequate follow up of the patient is advised.

401 A benign pedunculated polyp is seldom shown up in an ordinary barium enema and requires a double contrast enema of the Welin type as shown here.

402 This sessile polyp was associated with passage of blood per rectum and was in fact a carcinoma of colon.

403 Multiple polyposis of colon These are true polyps as opposed to the pseudopolyps in ulcerative colitis. In this case there was a family history of polyposis coli with a high incidence of carcinoma of colon. The large polyp in the centre is a carcinoma.

400

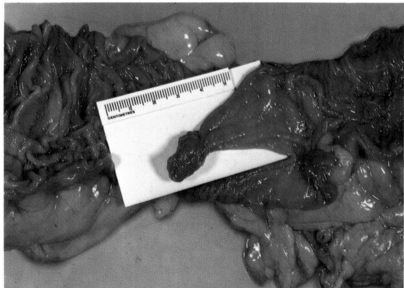

401

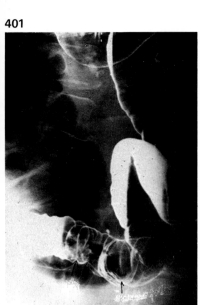

402

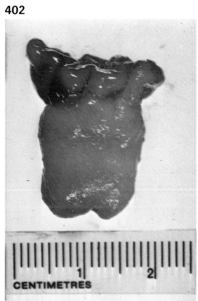

403

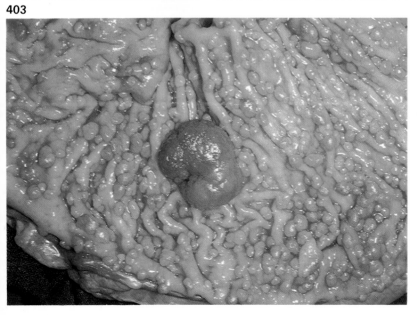

404 Parasitic infection of colon This histological section shows the presence of schistosoma in the wall of the bowel. It represents an important cause of diarrhoea in the tropics. There are, of course, many other causes of tropical diarrhoea.

404

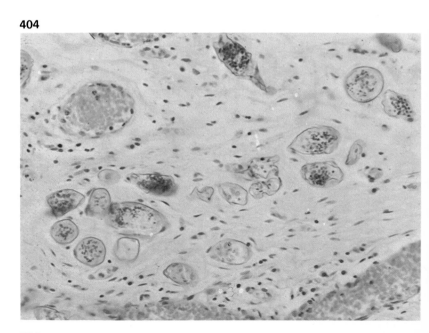

Cancer of colon

The signs and symptoms vary with the site of the tumour. In the right colon the symptoms are especially vague; a pain in right iliac fossa, anaemia, occult blood in faeces, and sensation of a mass. In the left colon the diagnostic features are a change in bowel habit, obstructive symptoms and frank blood in faeces. Rectal lesions also produce altered bowel habit, a feeling of something in the back passage and frank bleeding which may lead to the mistaken diagnosis of piles.

405 This carcinoma of caecum gave the vague symptoms described above. Barium enema using the double contrast techniques demonstrated the lesion.

405

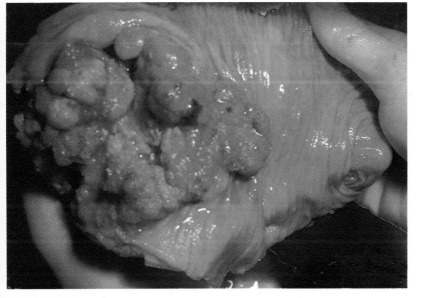

406 Small carcinoma of pelvic colon shown on the left was found in a patient who had a benign polyp removed two years previously. A change in bowel habit led to re-examination. A second polyp is shown on the right.

407 This small carcinoma just palpable on rectal examination as a small nodule was found in a patient with a massively enlarged liver due to secondaries.

408 Carcinoma of the rectum is often quite large before it is detected as the bleeding is usually put down to piles. This one is of more reasonable size.

409 This carcinoma of colon appeared in a bowel affected by a rather uncommon condition, melanosis coli. The association is quite fortuitous.

406

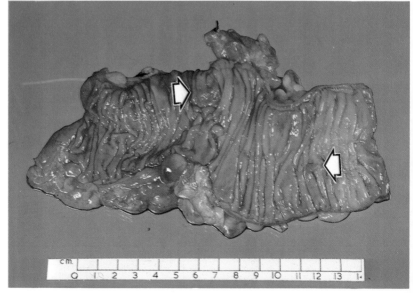

407

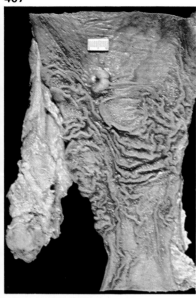

408

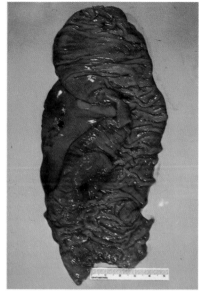

409

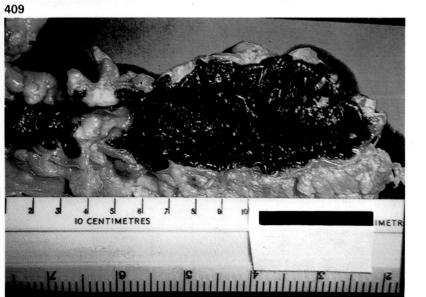

239

Ano-rectal lesions

410 Anal fissure gives rise to severe pain felt on passage of a large piece of faeces. Bleeding is common on defaecation. The fissure is seen at 6 o'clock.

411 Intero-external piles produce these bulbous swellings in the anal region. Bleeding is common on defaecation.

412 Prolapsed piles may strangulate and, as here, become gangrenous.

413 Fistula-in-ano This patient had recurrent peri-anal infection and fistula formed between the skin and rectum. A probe could be inserted along the tracts. He had Crohn's disease of the rectum. Other causes are chronic infection, tuberculosis, and carcinoma.

414 Prolapse of rectum usually occurs by itself but may be associated, as shown, with a vaginal prolapse. Incontinence is often present, and bleeding or discharge may be noted.

415 Ischio-rectal abscess is a very painful inflammatory lesion in the ischio-rectal fossa. The pain, redness and tenderness are diagnostic. Incision should be made before fluctuation – a late sign.

410

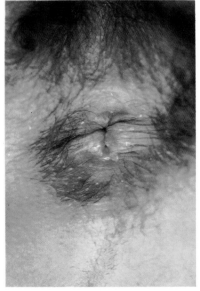

411

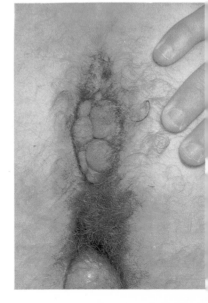

412

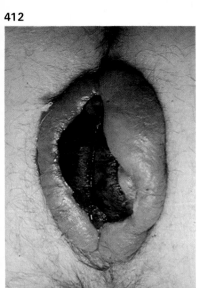

413

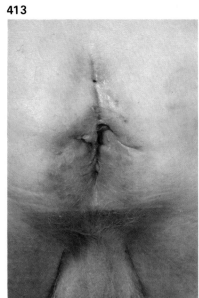

414

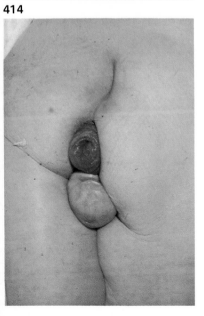

415

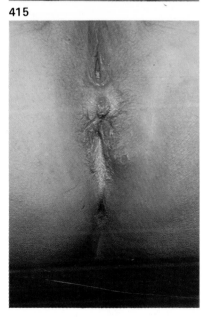

416 Tuberculosis of the anal canal is rare. It presents as a fistula-in-ano and perianal inflammation. Diagnosis depends on biopsy.

417 Crohn's disease may affect the anal region. A chronic granulomatous lesion is present with discharge and anal discomfort. Multiple fistula *(pepperbox perineum)* can develop. Diagnosis is by biopsy.

416

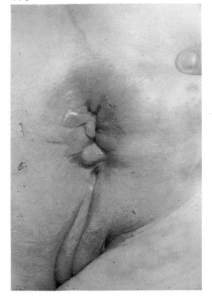

417

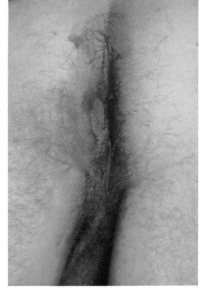

Tumours of anal canal and perineum

BENIGN TUMOURS (ANAL WARTS)

418 Anal warts, usually termed venereal warts, are of viral origin.

MALIGNANT TUMOURS

419 Squamous carcinoma presents the features of the lesion as seen on the skin elsewhere. They present with bleeding, discharge with soiling, pruritis, local pain, the feeling of a lump, and sometimes tenesmus. Biopsy will define the type of lesion present.

418

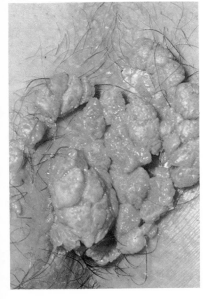

419

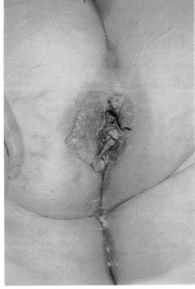

420 Basal cell carcinoma is not common. It presents similarly to **419**. Diagnosis is made on biopsy.

421 Basiloid carcinoma arises from embryologic remnants. The bulk of the tumour is in the deeper tissue with only the apex appearing in the anal canal. Biopsy is necessary to establish the diagnosis.

Miscellaneous

422 Imperforate anus No opening for meconium is visible in the perineum. The bowel ended blindly above the pubo-rectalis muscle. A plain x-ray shows the level of air in the bowel in relation to a skin marker.

423 A colostomy done to relieve an imperforate anus. It would probably have been better to have done a right transverse colostomy leaving the left side clear for definitive operation.

420

421

422

423

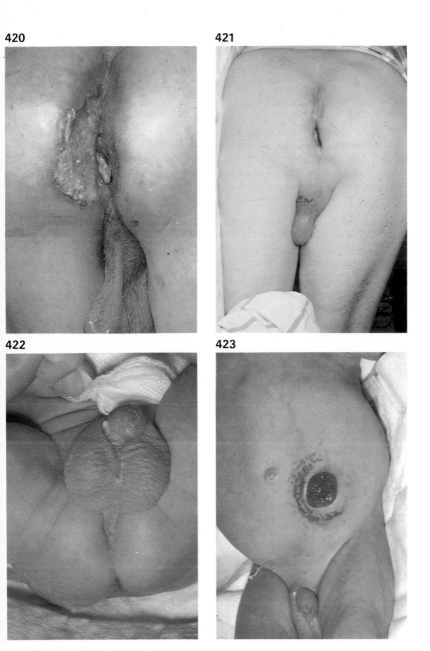

Disease of the Liver

424 Hepatomegaly is due to a variety of causes: infection, neoplasm, and metabolism. Diagnosis is based on history, clinical examination, radiography, liver function tests, haematology, bone marrow and liver biopsy and liver scan.

425 Chronic hepatitis with ascites This patient was thought to have malignant disease. Various tests were somewhat equivocal. Diagnosis was finally established by liver biopsy.

426 Liver abscess is usually pyogenic secondary to infection in alimentary tract or biliary system, but may be amoebic or parasitic. An enlarged tender liver with fever, rigors, and jaundice may suggest the diagnosis which is confirmed by signs of infection and the details of a liver scan. The abscesses shown here were secondary to diverticulitis.

424

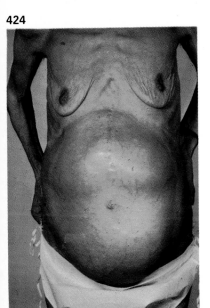

425

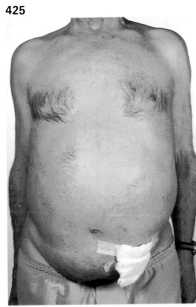

426

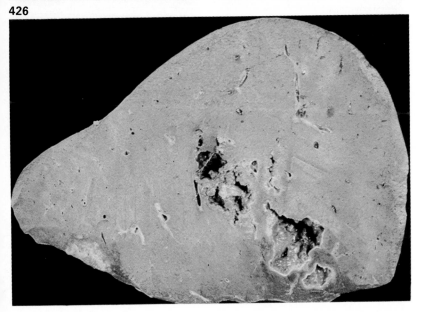

427 Hydatid cysts These cause hepatomegaly and a chronic pain in the right hypochondrium. They occur in endemic areas. Liver scan and selective angiography will outline the cysts. Immunological tests, haemagglutination inhibition and complement fixation tests are useful.

428 Hydatid cyst Aspiration and the injection of a scolicidal agent (formalin; phenol 20% saline) help to prevent anaphylaxis or implantation.

429 Hydatid cysts The common site is in the right lobe of the liver. There may be a single cyst or as here multiple.

427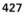

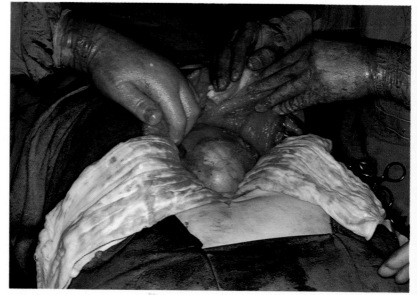

428

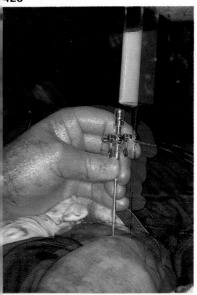

429

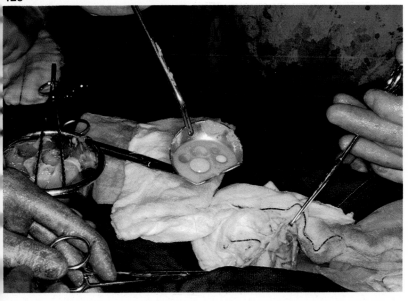

430 Cirrhosis of the liver may cause hepatomegaly with altered albumin/globulin ratio and possibly portal hypertension with splenomegaly and dilated oesophageal veins. These will be demonstrated on barium swallow or oesophagoscopy.

430

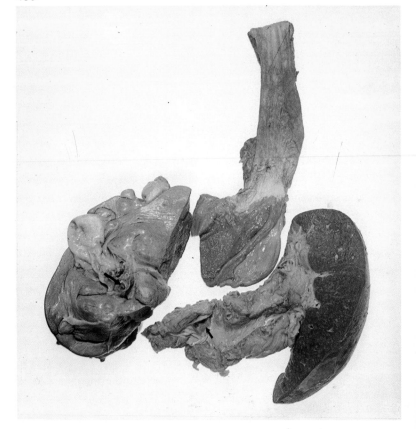

431 Cirrhosis of liver and portal hypertension. The patient presented with haematemesis. Albumin was 3.2g/100 ml. Oesophageal varices were seen on barium swallow and required a port-caval anastomosis as shown here.

431

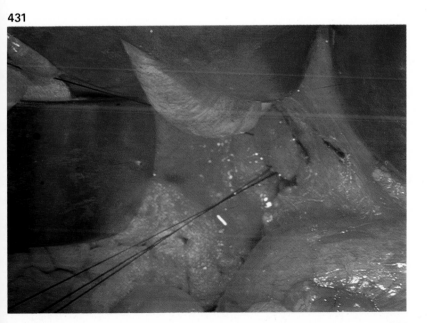

Tumours of the liver

These may, as elsewhere, be benign or malignant. The benign tumours are haemangioma and adenoma. Malignant tumours are nearly always secondary from breast, lung, pancreas, alimentary canal, ovary and uterus. The much less common primary tumours are hepatoma, cholangiocarcinoma, and in children the hepatoblastoma.

432 Benign adenoma shown here is associated with cirrhosis. The tumour is asymptomatic and very large.

433 Hepatoblastoma This occurred in a 22-month-old baby who presented with a huge mass in the abdomen. An I.V.P. excluded a renal tumour.

434 Hepatoblastoma removed with about 80% of the liver. The child survived the operation but died two years later with pulmonary metastases. The specimen is shown preserved.

432

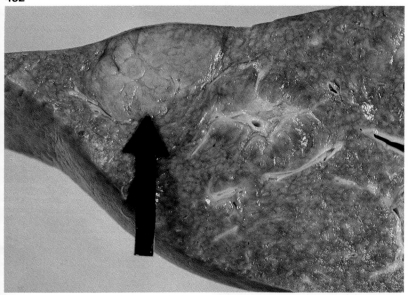

433

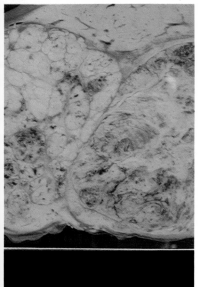

434

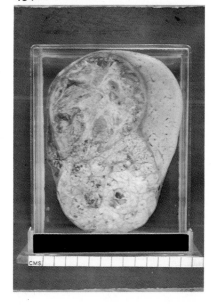

435 Hepatoblastoma Replacement of right lung by metastases from a hepatoblastoma. The child had increasing breathlessness and lassitude.

436 Hepatomas are often missed clinically. This five-year-old female patient had a vague upper abdominal pain and enlarging abdomen. The liver was enlarged. Liver scan showed that nearly the whole liver was involved. Angiography demonstrated the vascular pattern and a dense tumour blush.

437 The same hepatoma exposed at operation was found impossible to remove. Ligation of hepatic artery was carried out.

435

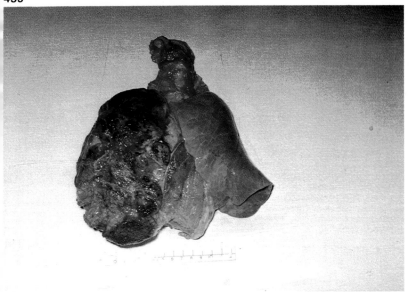

436

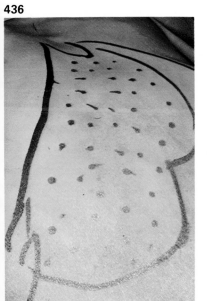

437

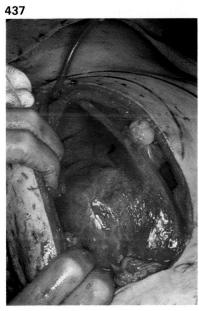

438 Pathological specimen of a primary hepatoma Fever, loss of
weight, jaundice, and bloody ascites supported the diagnosis. A positive
alpha-fetoprotein test is of diagnostic value.

439 A large hepatoma was found at post-mortem in this patient, known to
have cirrhosis. He suddenly began to deteriorate rapidly and ascites developed. Paracentesis revealed blood in the fluid.

440 This woman had jaundice and an enlarged liver Note no jaundice
in sclera of her right eye – it was a glass eye! The classical association is a
melanoma of an eye which is removed and later secondaries develop in the
liver. She had in fact a *cancer of the pancreas* and the glass eye was
incidental.

441 Hepatomegaly is often due to replacement of liver by secondary
neoplasm. The alkaline phosphatase is usually raised.

438

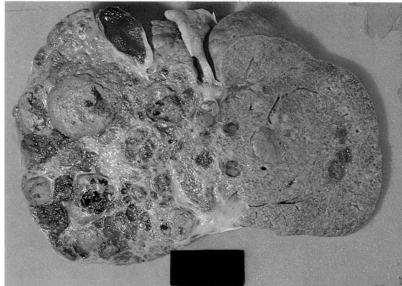

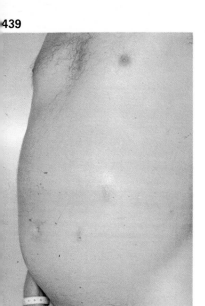

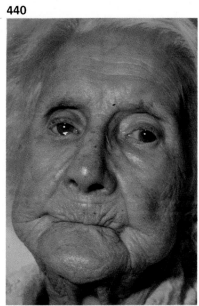

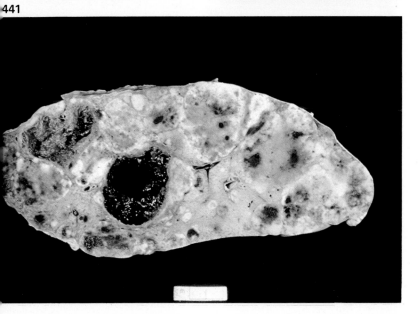

Disease of the Gallbladder

442 Gallstones are of three main types: pure cholesterol, as in the right of the second row: pure pigment (the black ones); and the mixed stones with varying colour patterns.

443 Jaundice presents a typical picture of yellow skin and conjunctiva. The problem is in the differentiation of the various causes: haemolytic, hepatic, and obstructive. This requires good history taking, examination and the use of many investigations.

444 A resected specimen of a choledochus cyst This rare condition of cystic dilatation of part or whole of the wall of the common bile duct presents usually in females as a swelling in the right hypochonrium with recurrent attacks of pain, jaundice, and pyrexia. An intravenous cholangiogram will help in the diagnosis.

442

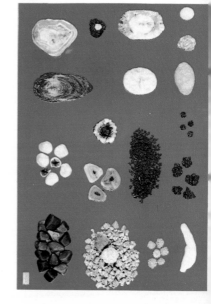

443

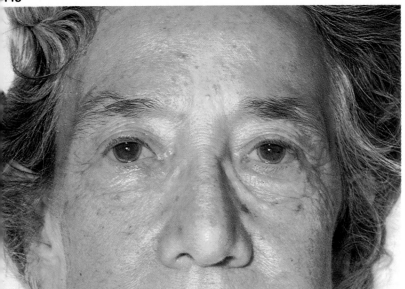

444

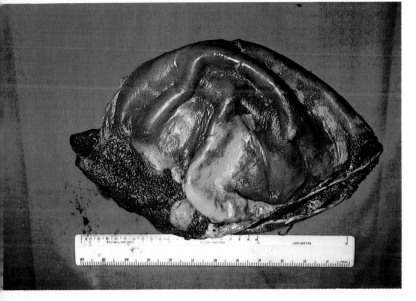

445 Acute cholecystitis presents with acute epigastric and right upper quadrant pain and tenderness under the subcostal margin at tip of 9th rib. Fever and leucocytosis are noted. The gallbladder may be felt in about 35% of patients. A nonfunctioning gallbladder will be reported after oral or intravenous cholangiogram.

446 Acute cholecystitis full of gallstones which extend down into Hartmann's pouch. It is the blockage of the cystic duct by gallstones that causes the vast majority of cases of this kind.

447 Gangrenous cholecystitis is suggested by continuation of the pain and fever despite treatment. The gallbladder may be much enlarged. Gangrene occurs earlier than empyema from which it is otherwise difficult to differentiate.

448 A mucocoele of the gallbladder occurs due to cystic duct obstruction without infection. The gallbladder is usually palpable and not really tender.

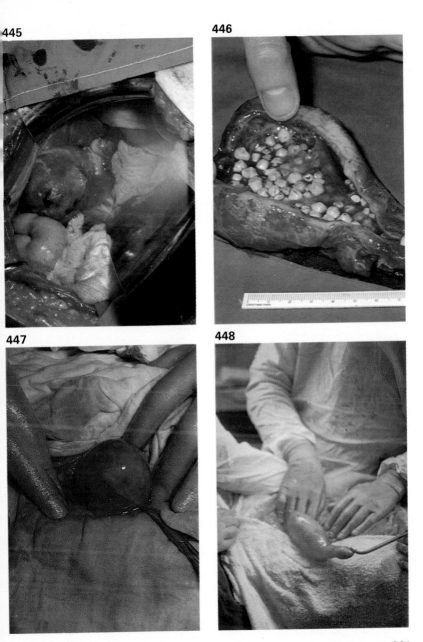

445

446

447

448

449 Chronic cholecystitis may be asymptomatic and found during investigation or operation. The symptoms are recurrent epigastric pain and dyspepsia which is classically of fatty type but may not be so. Gallstones may be visible on plain x-ray (20%) or on cholecystography.

450 Carcinoma of the gallbladder may appear like chronic cholecystitis or, if the cystic duct is obstructed by tumour, as an acute cholecystitis as in this patient. It is almost impossible to diagnose before operation.

451 Cancer of gallbladder The secondaries are seen scattered throughout the liver.

452 Carcinoma of the bile duct is uncommon and difficult to diagnose. This patient had a mild jaundice and the diagnosis was made on exploration for a stone in the duct or a cancer of head of pancreas.

449

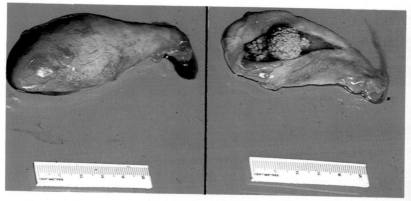

450

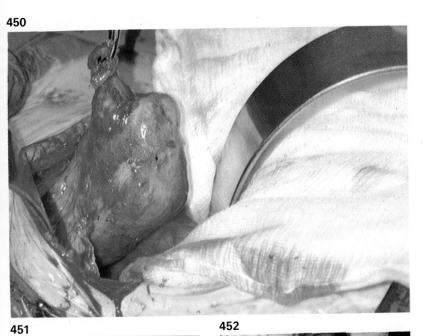

451

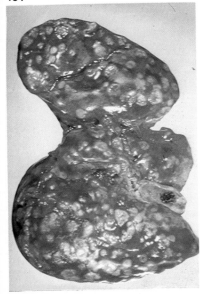

452

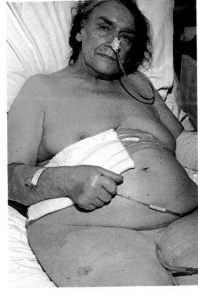

Disease of the Pancreas

453 Annular pancreas is a collar of pancreatic tissue surrounding the second part of the duodenum producing obstruction if the tissue is thick enough. Symptoms if present are those of duodenal obstruction. A plain x-ray may show a 'double-bubble' appearance.

454 Annular pancreas seen on x-ray of a baby with duodenal obstruction. The huge distended stomach is seen on the right and to the left the 'double bubble'.

455 Acute pancreatitis The post-mortem specimen is from a patient who died with acute haemorrhagic pancreatitis. He had sudden onset of severe epigastric pain passing through to the back. Nausea, vomiting and shock followed. He was tender all over the abdomen but especially in the epigastrum. The serum amylase was over 2,000 units.

456 Acute pancreatitis The lipase enzyme produces fat necrosis and with the formation of calcium soaps the serum calcium may fall.

457 Grey Turner's sign of acute pancreatitis is rare. It is a greenish discoloration in the left loin.

453

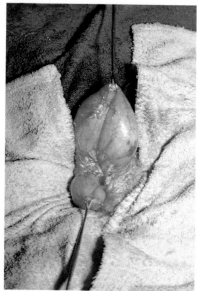

454

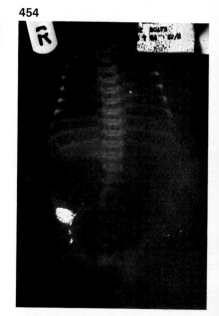

455

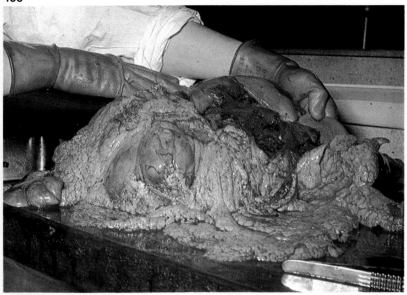

456

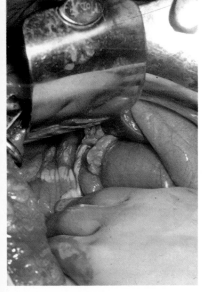

457

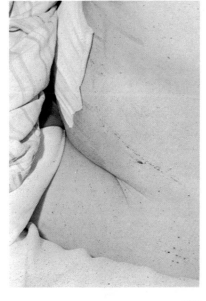

458 Umbilical discoloration (Cullen's sign) may be seen in acute pancreatitis similar to that described by Cullen in a ruptured ectopic gestation. The bluish greenish discoloration is due to the action of pancreatic ferments on the subcutaneous tissue producing a haemorrhagic necrosis.

459 Chronic pancreatitis is characterised by recurrent attacks of epigastric pain radiating to the back. Some patients develop malabsorption with steatorrhoea, others diabetes. This specimen was removed because of severe attacks occurring almost weekly. The gallbladder had been removed previously. The secretion test showed a low bicarbonate secretion.

460 A pancreatogram was carried out at operation in the previous case, by inserting a tube into the duct after resecting the tail of the pancreas. Radio-opaque material was injected and a film taken to demonstrate presence of strictures of the duct.

458

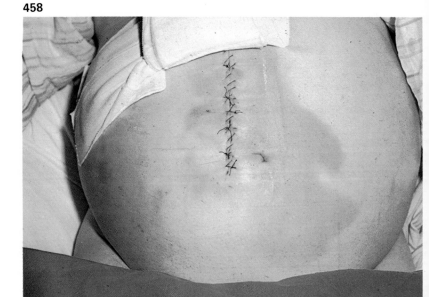

459

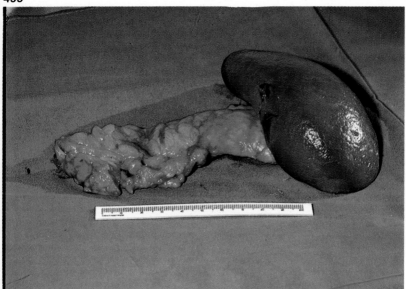

460

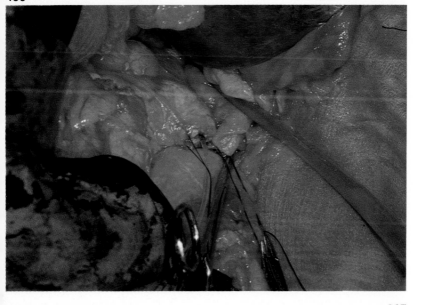

267

461 Pseudocysts of pancreas are collections of fluid usually in the lesser sac enclosed in a fibrous capsule. They may follow pancreatitis or trauma. The clinical features are persistent epigastric pain, and epigastric mass. A barium meal may show displacement of the stomach.

462 Pseudocyst of pancreas This shows a barium meal after treatment of the cyst by anastamosis to back of the stomach. It shows the size and extension of the cyst.

463 Pancreatic fistula This followed the drainage of a pancreatic abscess near the tail of the pancreas. The fluid contained pancreatic ferment.

464 Pancreatic fistula A close up view of **463** shows the clear fluid being extruded. The cyst was cleaned up finally by anastomosis of the end of the fistula into a loop of jejunum.

461

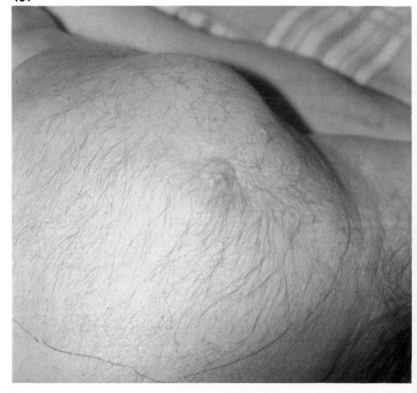

462

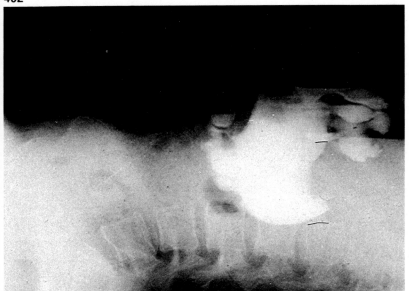

463

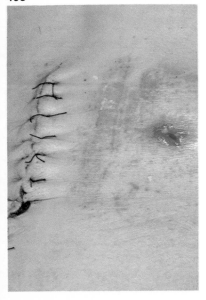

464

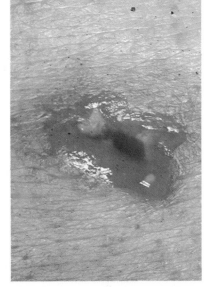

Tumours of the pancreas

Clinical features

Non-endocrine

Adenocarcinoma	Painless progressive jaundice, later pain, loss of weight, mass
Cystadenoma	Pain and mass
Cystadenocarcinoma	Pain and mass

Endocrine

Insulinoma	Whipple's triad
Gastrinoma	Zollinger-Ellison syndrome
Glucagonoma	Hyperglycaemia
Non-islet cell adenoma	Watery diarrhoea: hypokalaemia

465 Carcinoma of pancreas The typical picture in an elderly person with a progressive jaundice. The adenocarcinoma arises usually in the head of the pancreas. Epigastric pain and loss of weight are features. A barium meal will demonstrate expansion of the duodenum. The gallbladder may be large and non-tender. This plus jaundice is Courvoisier's sign.

466 Islet-cell tumour of the pancreas causes attacks of hypoglycaemia relieved by ingestion of food. Whipple's triad is classical hypoglycaemic symptoms with a fasting blood glucose below 50mg/100 ml and relief of the symptoms by administration of glucose.

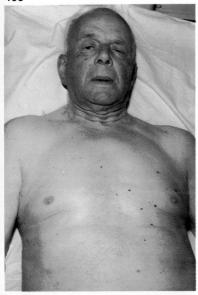

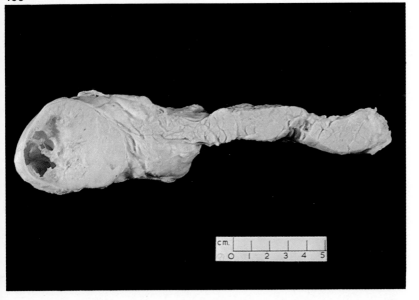

467 Splenomegaly is not usually as gross as this in the western world. The swelling was smooth with an anterior border outlined in blue. It extends left to the costal margin and above. The upper end cannot therefore be defined. On respiration the swelling moves down on inspiration. The circle marks the greatest depth of the spleen.

467

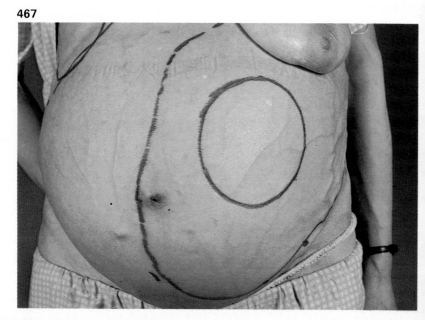

468 The splenomegaly in this young woman produced hypersplenism. She was found to have chronic leukaemia. The other main causes of such a marked splenomegaly in Britain are polycythaemia and portal hypertension. In tropical countries protozoal infection is a more likely cause.

468

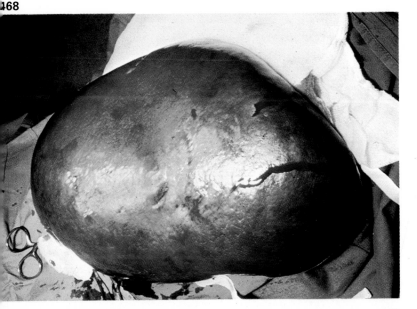

Abdominal Injuries

Abdominal injuries may occur alone or with injuries in other parts of the body which overshadow the abdominal lesion.

Clinical features The three main features are abdominal pain, tenderness, and distension. Peristalsis may be absent or diminished. Bleeding may be intra-peritoneal. Haematemesis, haematuria or melaena may accompany shock.

Investigations Plain x-ray will show lower rib fractures which point to injury of liver or spleen. Pneumoperitoneum indicates rupture of intestine. Intravenous pyelogram and possibly cystoscopy or cystography may be indicated if haematuria is present. Abdominal parcentesis is usually done as a four quadrant tap and may show presence of blood or bile.

469 Liver injury may be minor with minimal signs or massive with severe shock, abdominal pain, and tenderness all over but most marked in the liver area. Pain may be felt in the right shoulder and on x-ray the lower ribs on the right side may show fractures.

470 Splenic injury The classic features are, a blow on the left lower chest or upper abdomen with possibly a fracture of ribs, abdominal pain beginning in left hypochondrium and in time spreading throughout the abdomen and pain in the left shoulder *(Kehr's sign)*. Splenic dullness may be increased and tenderness will be noted over ninth rib on left side. Splenic rupture often has minimal signs to begin with and delayed collapse may occur hours or even days later.

471 Splenic injury The patient with this transected spleen collapsed immediately after injury and was severely shocked on admission to hospital. About three pints of blood were sucked out of the peritoneal cavity.

472 Splenic injury This spleen with the surrounding haematoma was removed from a woman injured in a traffic accident. She had other injuries which required urgent treatment. The splenic rupture was missed. A week later she suddenly collapsed and had an obvious intraperitoneal bleeding. At operation the left hypochondrium was full of old clot. Fresh bleeding had occurred prior to the collapse.

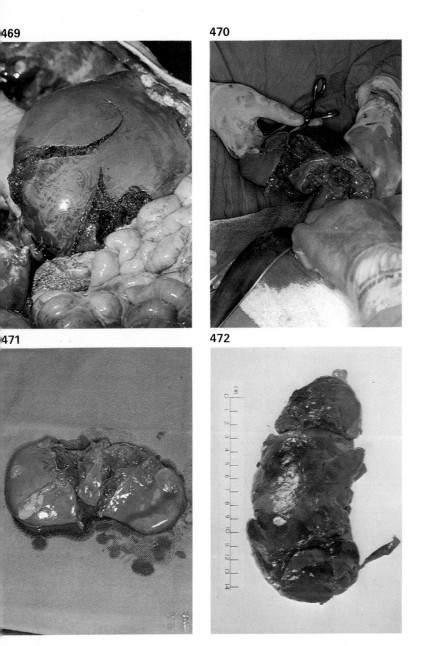

469

470

471

472

473 Renal injury The laceration of the kidney was due to blunt trauma. The patient collapsed shortly thereafter and on catheterisation of the bladder fresh blood was found. An emergency I.V.P. showed a leakage of contrast material into the surrounding area. At operation the bleeding had extended to produce a mesenteric haematoma.

474 Renal injury due to gunshot wound The entry of a 0.22 bullet can be seen at the lateral end of the transection wound. The damaged kidney was found on exploration of the bullet wound in a collapsed patient.

475 Rupture of a pathological kidney may occur from a relatively minor injury. This hydronephrotic kidney was removed from a young student who fell playing football. The injury was minor but he complained of severe pain in the left loin. Haematuria was present. I.V.P. confirmed rupture of kidney. The hydronephrosis was previously unsuspected.

473

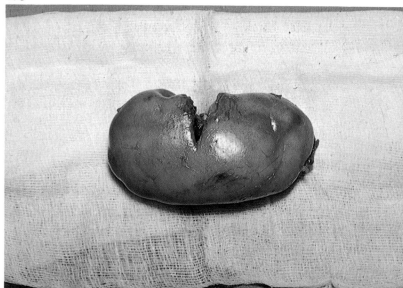

474

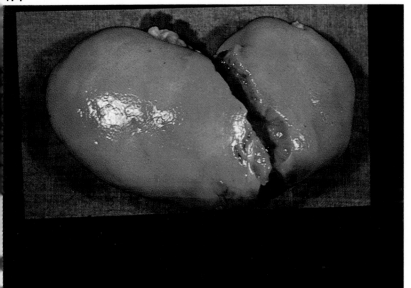

475

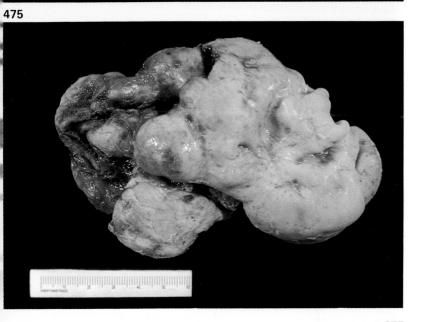

476 Extravasation of urine produces a characteristic picture of extension of a brawny oedema above the pubis, into penis, and down into the thigh.

477 Extraperitoneal rupture of the bladder is demonstrated here by the forceps. This lesion is not common but can occur with pelvic injuries and may be missed initially if catheterisation is not carried out. Confirmation can be obtained from cystography or cystoscopy.

478 Rupture of bowel This perforation of the jejuneum occurred about 20 cms from the duodeno-jejunal flexure. It was caused by blunt trauma in a patient involved in a road traffic accident. A pneumoperitoneum was present on plain x-ray.

476

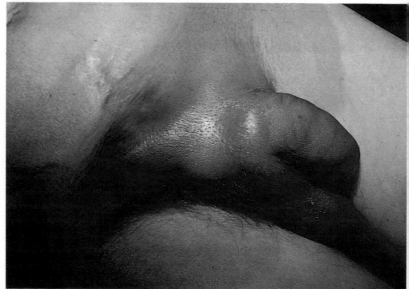

477

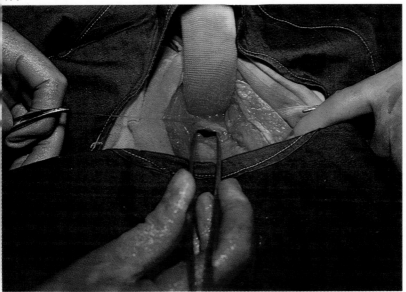

478

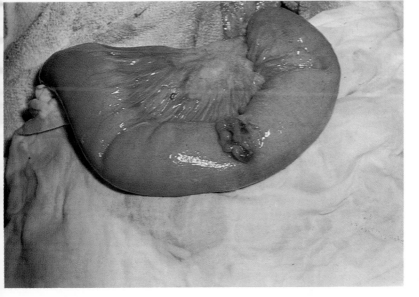

479 Late perforation of small bowel with peritonitis. This was found in a patient who complained of sudden abdominal pain, nausea and vomiting. There was no obvious cause for the perforation. The patient had received a blow on the abdomen five days previously but this had passed almost unnoticed.

480 Stab wound of abdomen This type of injury is sometimes seen in butchers using a boning knife. It may damage the femoral artery. In this patient the knife passed upwards and perforation of colon had to be excluded by exploration.

481 A tear in the mesentery may follow blunt trauma and the bleeding may be sufficient to cause death. The mesentary is crushed against the vertebrae. A needle tap would show the presence of blood in the peritoneal cavity.

479

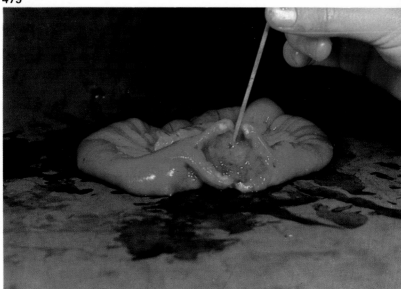

480

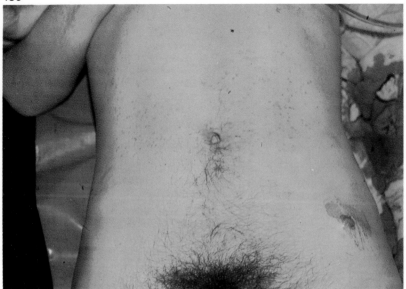

481

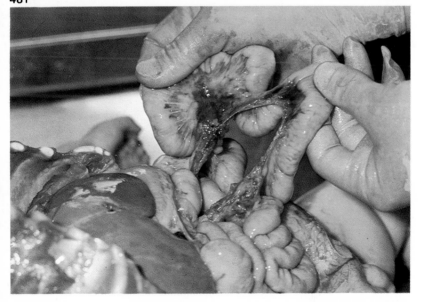

Disease of the Breast

482 A supernumerary nipple is sometimes seen along a line extending from normal breast area to the groin. It should not be confused with a simple skin tumour.

483 Mastitis of infancy is a hypertrophy of breast tissue due to excess of hormone from the mother. A milky secretion may be expressed from the nipple – 'witch's milk'. A similar condition may also be seen at puberty.

484 Inversion of the nipple may have been present since puberty, when it is of no significance. If it is of recent origin in adult life one should examine for a scirrhous carcinoma. If no lump is palpable consider mammography, xeroradiography or thermography to exclude an early lesion.

482

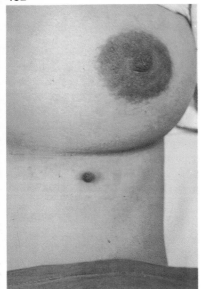

483

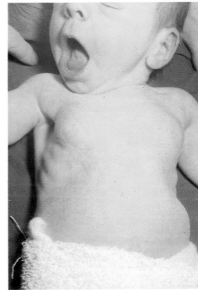

484

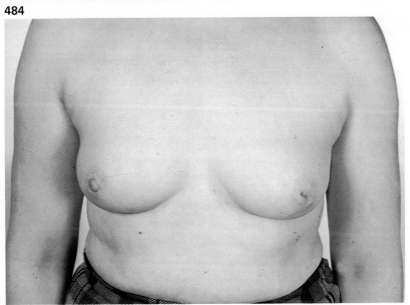

485 A blood-stained discharge from the nipple signifies the presence of a duct papilloma or carcinoma. Pressure on different areas of the breast may localise the probable site. Other discharges from the nipple are milky *(lactation),* clear serous *(retention cyst),* black or green *(chronic mastitis)* and purulent *(breast abscess).*

486 Breast abscess in the lactating breast is usually due to the staphylococcus. The clinical features of the acute inflammation are classical unless antibiotics have been given at an early stage. This may produce a chronic granuloma or abscess which might be mistaken for carcinoma.

487 Breast abscess in the non-lactating breast is rare and when it does occur is usually a subareolar abscess. In this patient the abscess was exactly similar to that in the lactating breast. It is important not to wait for fluctuation to occur as this is a late sign associated with massive breast destruction.

485

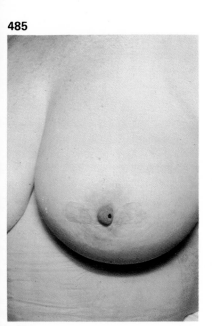

486

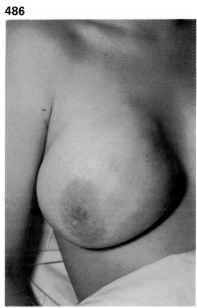

487

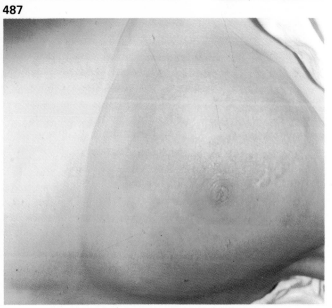

488 Chronic mastitis (mammary dysplasia; fibroadenosis) This common condition occurs in women aged 30–50. There is pain in the breasts especially at the period time. If diffuse there is a nodular rubbery feel to both breasts. Localised areas are felt as indefinite lumps, rubbery and tender. When palpating with the flat of the hand against the chest wall the lump disappears in contrast to a cancer. No nodes are felt. The specimen shows the fibrosis and cystic change.

489 Cyst of breast shown here being aspirated is most commonly associated with other conditions. The cyst is felt as a smooth rounded cystic area in a nodular breast. The fluid aspirated may be clear as here.

490 Further aspiration in another cyst shows the greenish content. The cysts are commonly multiple and small. In any area of breast removed for chronic mastitis a number of tiny cysts may be seen. If the fluid aspirated is bloody then excision biopsy should be done to exclude cancer.

488

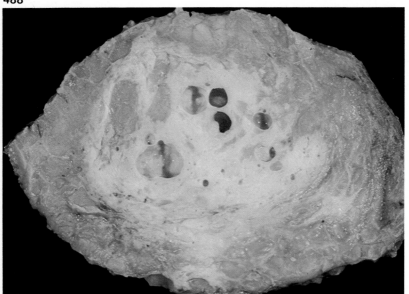

489

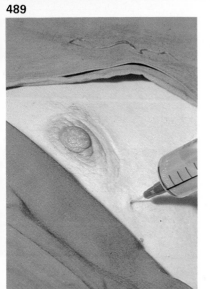

490

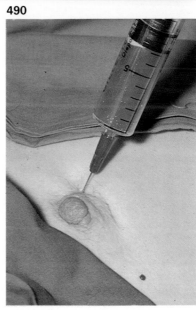

491 Fibroadenoma of breast is a common benign neoplasm found in young women. The lump is smooth, firm and mobile. Its firm nature can be well seen here. Two types of breast fiboadenomas exist; the hard, described here, and the rare soft variety which occurs in older women.

492 Cystosarcoma phylloides (serocystic disease of Brodie) is a type of soft fibroadenoma which grows quickly and may attain a large size. The bosselated surface, large size, firm and soft even cystic areas, and mobility are characteristics.

493 Another example of cystosarcoma phylloides which is not as malignant as its name suggests. Indeed it is usually regarded as being benign. Malignant change can however occur in roughly 20% of cases. In this patient the tumour was not unlike a fungating carcinoma except for mobility and absence of glands.

491

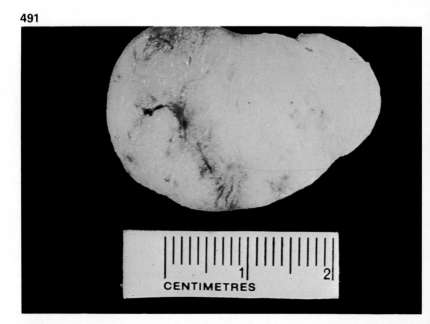

492

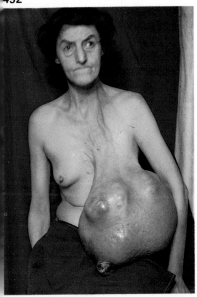

493

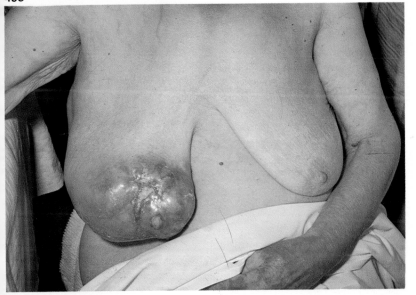

494 Intraduct papilloma is an uncommon lesion. It presents as a blood-stained discharge from the nipple. It is small and soft and may be impalpable, but if large can be felt as a mass near the nipple. Pressure on the mass causes the discharge from the nipple.

495 Paget's disease This shows an eczematous condition of the areola and erosion of the nipple, Paget's disease; a large mass in the breast and elevation of the nipple, indicative of cancer, and redness of the skin seen with a relatively uncommon type of cancer, mastitis carcinosa.

496 Paget's disease The eczematous condition has spread beyond the areola on to the skin of breast. The presence of an underlying tumour mass can be appreciated.

497 Paget's disease A close up view shows that the condition is not merely an eczema but the raised red tissue suggests infiltration of the areola due to the slowly growing underlying cancer.

494

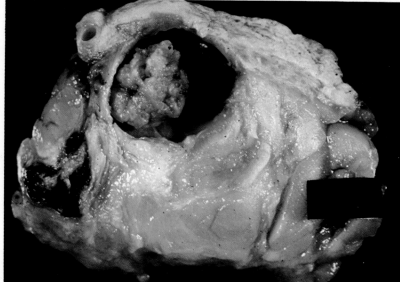

495

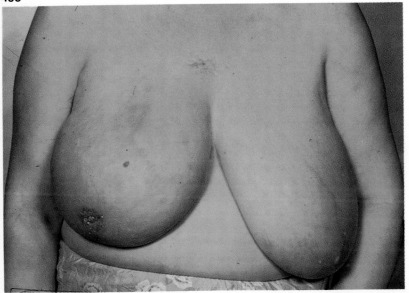

496

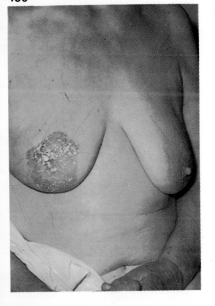

497

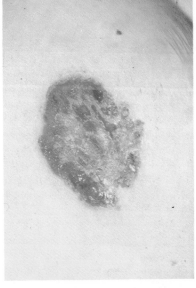

498 Cancer of breast This section of an anaplastic or medullary cancer of the breast seen as a round area in the centre of the picture illustrates that the early findings are a single, nontender, firm to hard mass in a woman over 45 years of age. The anaplastic tumour is seen at a younger age than the scirrhous type.

499 Cancer of breast The single mobile mass in the patient was accompanied by the important sign nipple retraction. The mass lies between the fingers. No glands were palpable. On cut section the mass was more ill defined than the previous one and was typical of a scirrhous carcinoma.

500 Peau d'orange is a classic late sign of cancer of the breast and usually is seen in advanced cancer. The peau d'orange is made more obvious by finger pressure. It is due to lymphatic oedema. The pits represent the fixed opening of the sweat ducts which cannot expand with oedema.

498

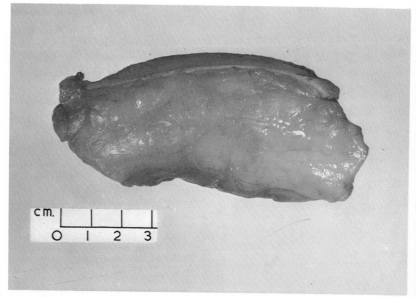

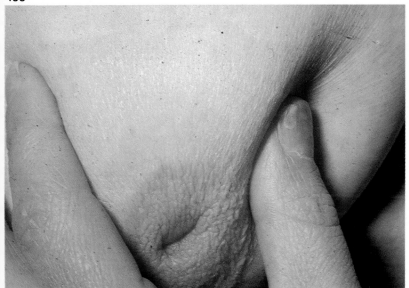

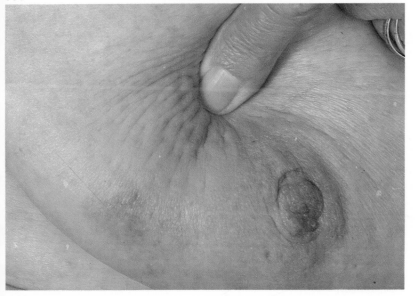

501 Peau d'orange In the large cancer of the breast there is a suspicion of peau d'orange in the lower half of the breast.

502 Peau d'orange The suspicion in **501** is confirmed by pressure of the finger.

503 Cancer of breast in the male is rare but even more dangerous because involvement of muscle and skin in a small breast is rapid. In this patient the tumour has ulcerated and spread to glands in the axilla.

501

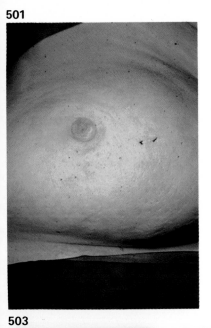

502

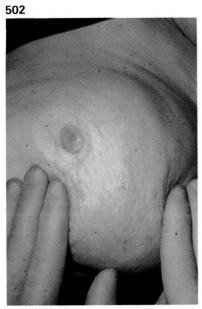

503

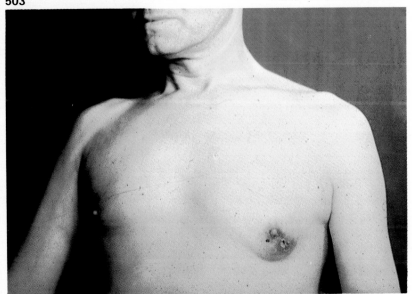

504 Lymphoedema of the arm This is usually seen years after a radical mastectomy especially if accompanied by x-ray therapy. It may however be seen, as here, in a patient with an extensive tumour which has blocked the lymphatics in the axilla.

505 Fungating cancer of breast Fungation is accompanied here by extensive skin metastases spreading up into the neck and across to the other breast.

506 Mastitic carcinosa or inflammatory carcinoma is a rare but very malignant form of breast cancer. The clinical features are a rapidly growing mass in the breast, the overlying skin is red, warm and sometimes oedematous.

504

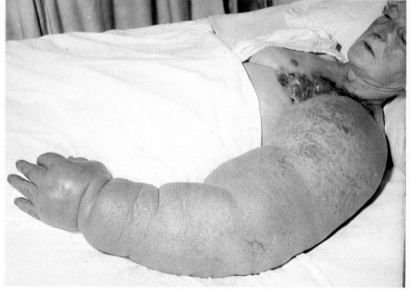

505

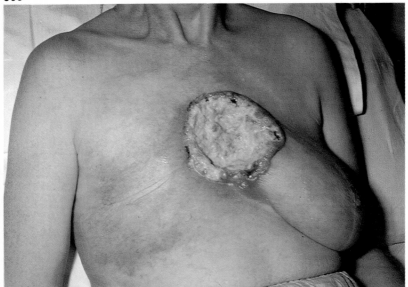

506

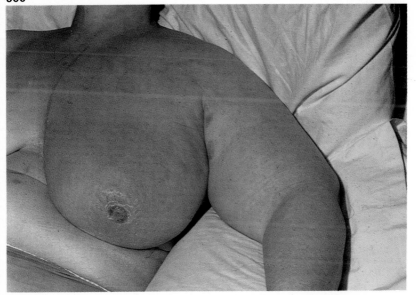

507 An atrophic scirrhous cancer is seen in the aged. Although this old lady had the tumour for five years there was no glandular involvement in the axilla.

508 Fungating cancer This has occurred in a patient with a previous right mastectomy. The lesion has probably come from a skin secondary. It does raise the question of another tumour in the other breast which is said to occur in about eight per cent of cases.

509 Cancer en cuirasse This patient had a right mastectomy. A few years later a very extensive secondary spread appeared involving the whole of the anterior chest wall in a fixed mass of tissue. Bilateral lymphoedema of the arms is present.

507

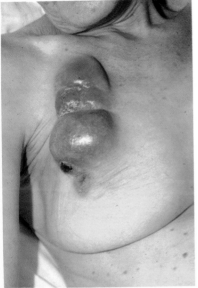

508

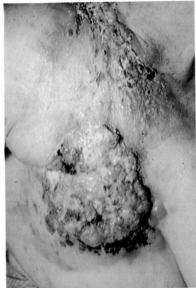

509

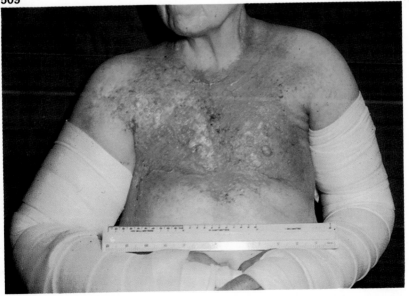

299

Renal Lesions

Developmental abnormalities

Due to the complex development of the kidney from the three primary structures (*pronephros, mesonephros* and *metanephros*) and the failure of these to join properly, a variety of abnormalities may develop. Some of these are illustrated.

510 Polycystic kidney presents in the infant as an enlarging mass – unilateral or bilateral. This child had a large right renal swelling which was ballotable from front to rear and showed changes on I.V.P.

511 Polycystic kidneys The cysts may remain small for years or gradually increase in size to destroy the normal tissue. This patient died from renal failure. Both kidneys were massively involved.

512 Polycystic kidney sometimes declares itself by renal infection and haematuria. It is obviously important to have an I.V.P. not only for diagnosis but to make sure the other kidney is normal.

510

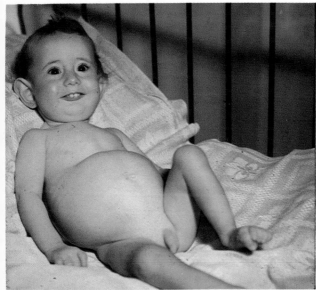

511

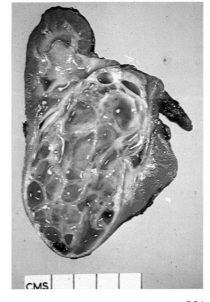

512

513 Unilocular cyst of kidney This lady noticed a gradual increase in the size of her abdomen and had discomfort in the left loin. The large swelling felt cystic and was easily ballotable. I.V.P. confirmed the lesion as being a renal cyst.

514 Unilocular cyst of kidney resected from the patient in **513**. Nephrectomy was carried out as there was very little function and the other kidney was normal. Renal arteriography can be done to differentiate between a cyst and tumour.

515 Unilocular cyst of kidney It was found possible to enucleate this cyst. Another technique is to aspirate with a needle especially under x-ray control. The aspirate is examined for blood and malignant cells.

516 Ectopic kidney A kidney may be fused or arrested at some stage in its ascent from the pelvic area. In this example the kidney lies in the right iliac fossa with its arterial supply coming from the right common iliac artery. This is the type of arteriogram we might expect in a transplanted kidney.

513

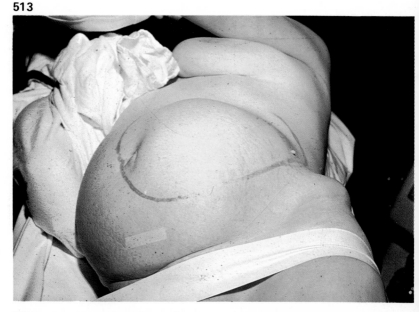

514

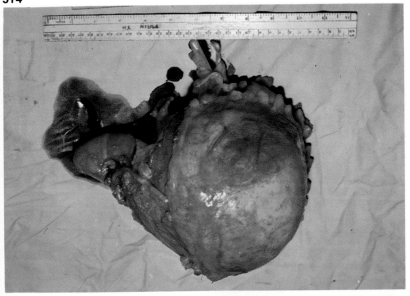

515

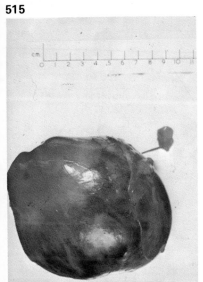

516

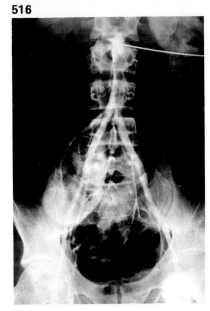

517 Double ureters are not uncommon and are seen on I.V.P. Of themselves they are of little consequence. The specimen was resected because there is an incidental carcinoma of renal pelvis.

518 Mobile kidney This is probably not congenital but more likely to be due to a reduction in perinephric fat. The right kidney is very low in position *(nephroptosis)*. The patient had intermittent attacks of pain in the left loin relieved by lying down *(Dietl's crisis)*. This is due to kinking of the ureter producing an early hydronephrosis.

517

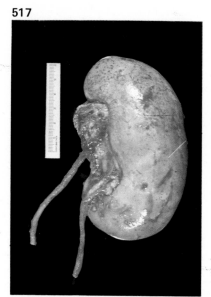

518

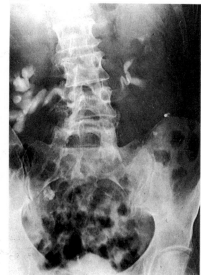

Obstructive nephropathy

A hydronephrosis is an aseptic dilatation of the kidney due to intermittent or partial obstruction of the urine outflow. It may be unilateral or bilateral and of congenital or acquired origin.

If the obstruction is at or distal to the bladder outlet the hydronephrosis is bilateral. If at or proximal to ureteric orifice then unilateral hydronephrosis will develop, unless both ureters are involved.

Clinical features These vary according to the site of obstruction. Renal hydronephrosis may be asymptomatic. If infection supervenes then frequency, dysuria and/or haematuria may occur. The kidney may be palpable, ballotable, and if infected or markedly distended, tender. An I.V.P. will confirm the diagnosis if there is any function in the affected kidney. Also, and very important, it will show the state of the other kidney. A full urological and laboratory work up is essential.

519 Bilateral hydronephrosis and hydroureter due to urethral valves in an infant. Death was by renal failure. Diagnosis was made at post-mortem examination in this case. Urethroscopy, cystoscopy and urethrography would have been helpful.

519

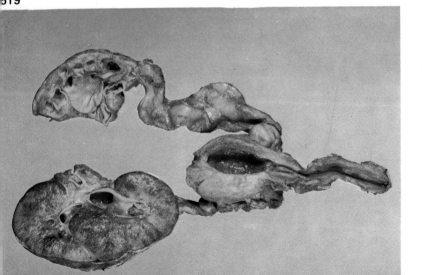

520 Hydronephrosis – unilateral This cross section of the kidney was obtained from a student whose kidney was ruptured by trauma. The presence of the hydronephrosis was unsuspected. The other kidney was normal on I.V.P.

521 Hydronephrosis due to neuromuscular inco-ordination at the pelvi-ureteric junction. The ureter is normal. The urine cannot be propelled adequately from renal pelvis into ureter.

522 Hydronephrosis A close up view of the pelvi-ureteric junction is shown with the narrow area which acts like an achalasia.

520

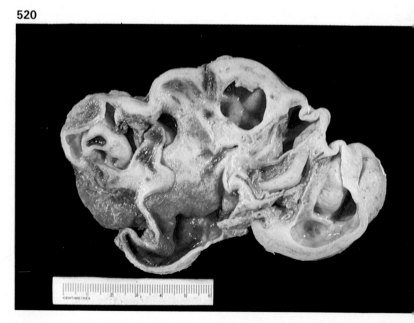

521

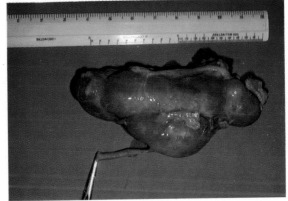

522

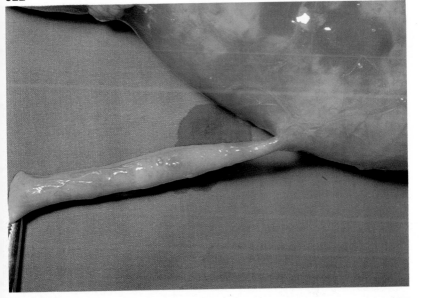

523 Hydronephrosis This lady had no previous trouble until seen with pain in the left loin and clinical features of urinary infection. A ballotable mass (outlined) was felt in the left loin.

524 Hydronephrosis The resected specimen of congenital hydronephrosis is shown with the catheter in the ureter. There is practically no renal cortex left.

525 Hydronephrosis with hypertension This kidney was resected from a man with a systolic blood pressure of 200 mmHg. After operation the pressure returned to a normal figure of 130 mmHg. This is an unusual feature of the hydronephrosis but nevertheless very welcome when it responds.

523

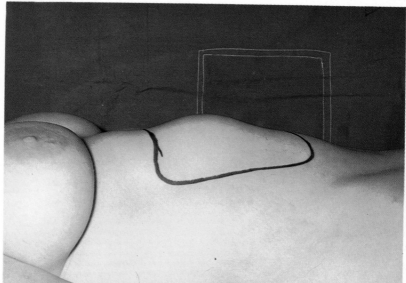

524

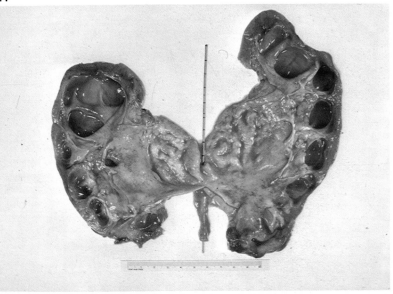

525

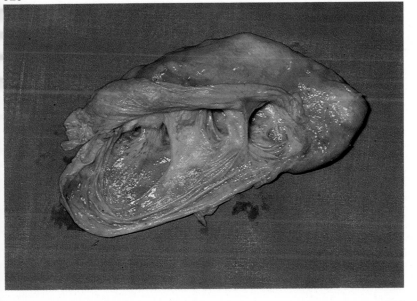

526 Hydronephrosis with aberrant renal vessel A gross pelvic
hydronephrosis is present. A tissue forceps is pulling on the hydronephrotic
kidney. The black silk suture is around the aberrant renal vessel and pulling it
away from the pelvi-ureteric junction. Although mentioned as a possible
cause of the hydronephrosis it is now commonly accepted as being incidental.

527 Hydronephrosis with aberrant renal artery This is an arteriogram
of the same patient, done as part of the investigation of hypertension.

526

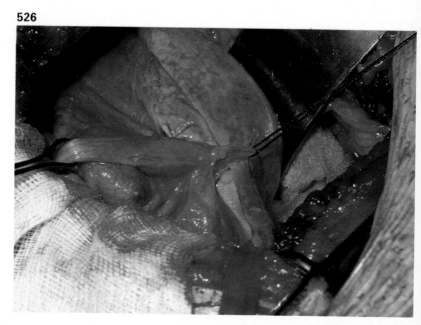

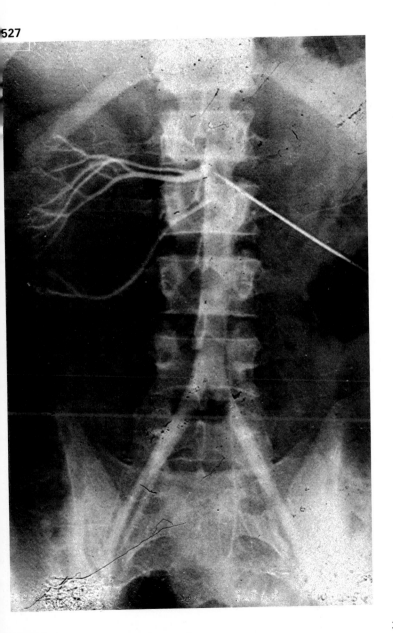

Urinary tract infection

There are two types of infection of the urinary tract: the common non-specific infection and the less common tuberculosis.

NON-SPECIFIC URINARY INFECTION

This is very common in surgical practice, indeed it is said to be the second most common type of infection in the human. The clinical features are loin or lower abdominal pain, frequency, dysuria, pyrexia with chills. In chronic infection, especially in the kidney, there may be no recognisable symptoms. Diagnosis is based on the clinical features, presence of tenderness, examination of the urine and I.V.P. Cystography may be necessary to reveal ureteric reflux.

528 Pyelonephritis may be acute or chronic. This specimen was removed from a patient who had recurrent urinary infection, a high blood pressure, and a very poorly functioning kidney on I.V.P. The other kidney looked normal.

528

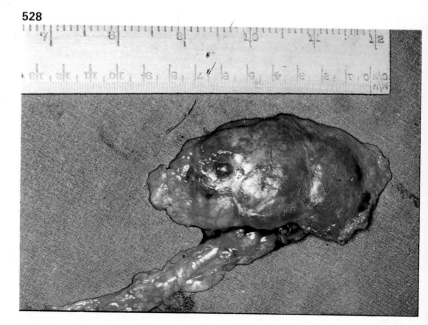

TUBERCULOSIS OF URINARY SYSTEM

This is less common now, but as it is commonly missed one should be on the look-out for it especially where there is pyuria without bacteriuria or a urinary tract infection which does not respond to treatment. The kidneys and epididymis are most commonly involved.

529 Renal tuberculosis The I.V.P. shows caliectasis of the right major calyx. Calcification was not present. Culture of the urine and guinea pig innoculation confirmed the presence of tuberculosis.

530 Renal tuberculosis This specimen was removed from a young woman with unilateral renal tuberculosis. The ureter and pelvis are dilated. The renal cortex is thinned and bulging due to scarring and internal softening and hydronephrotic change. Caseation is present in the lower pole.

529

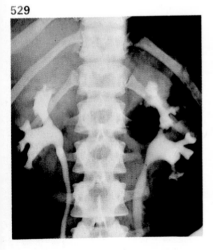

530

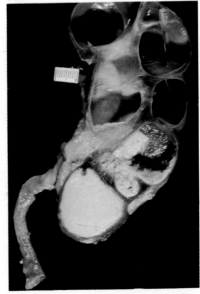

Renal stones

These are composed of the precipitated solid matter in the urine. The most common stones are phosphates, oxalates and urates. Others are uric acid, carbonates, cystine, leucine, and xanthine.

Clinical features are pain in the loin, haematuria, renal tenderness, and if infection presents, the signs of this. If stones obstruct the pelvic ureteric junction or pass into the ureter, then colic will occur. If no infection or obstruction is present then the stones may be asymptomatic. Diagnosis is confirmed by plain x-ray (80% positive) and I.V.P. Serum calcium and phosphorus should be estimated to exclude hyperparathyroidism.

531 Staghorn calculus These may develop to a large size gradually eroding the renal cortex. They may be unilateral or bilateral and cause loin pain. Urinary infection is often present and haematuria may occur.

532 Ureteric stone This is shown up in I.V.P. as a round space-filling lesion with proximal obstruction. The patient had severe colic.

533 Ureteric stone from the same patient displayed at operation.

534 Ureteric stone being extruded through the opened ureter.

531

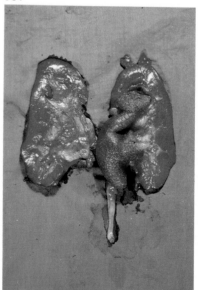

532

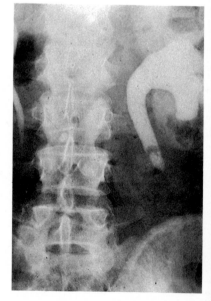

533

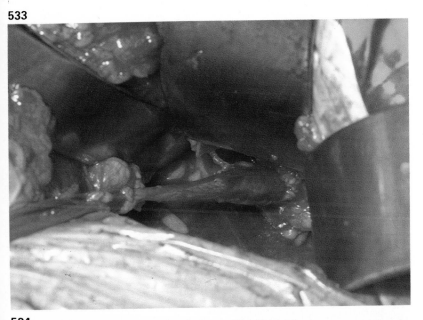

534

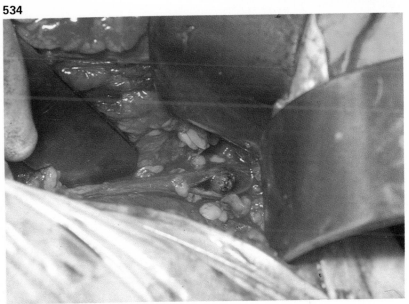

Tumours of kidney

BENIGN TUMOURS are rare. The commonest one is the adenoma which is found incidentally at post mortem examination. Fibroma, angioma and lipoma may also occur.

535 Benign adenoma of kidney Asymptomatic during life. Found at post mortem.

MALIGNANT TUMOURS of kidney are unfortunately common.

Clinical features The commonest symptom is painless haematuria. On examination the kidney may be palpable, and contain a mass. Renal pain is not a feature. Sometimes symptoms arise from metastases alone, e.g. pain in bones, loss of weight, and pulmonary complications.

Diagnosis is confirmed by I.V.P. and renal arteriography.

Classification

Primary	Secondary
Tubular carcinoma (Hypernephroma, Grawitz)	Carcinoma (bronchus, breast)
Nephroblastoma (Wilm's)	Melanoma
Renal pelvis – transitional cell cancer, squamous cancer	Lymphoma

536 Adenocarcinoma of kidney (hypernephroma) arising in upper pole. Patient had haematuria and on examination a large mass was found in the loin.

537 Adenocarcinoma of kidney The transected specimen demonstrates how the calyces in the lower part are compressed and would be visualised as such on I.V.P.

535

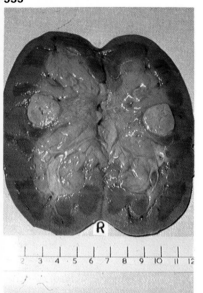

536

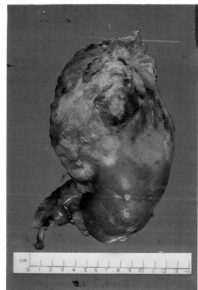

537

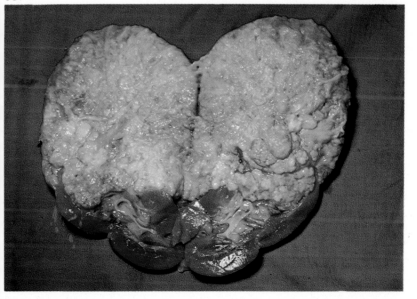

538

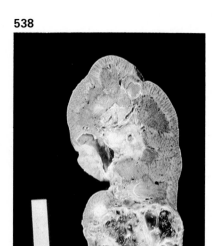

539

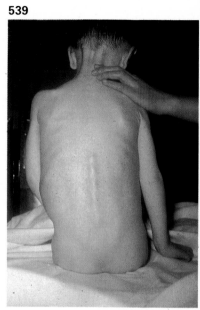

540

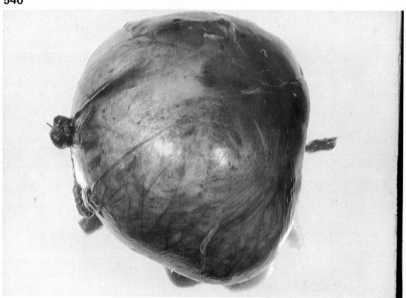

538 Adenocarcinoma of kidney demonstrating the haemorrhagic necrosis and degeneration that can take place due to the vascular nature of the tumour. On arteriography the whole area would be a mass of vascular tissue.

539 Nephroblastoma (Wilm's tumour) This 8-year-old boy was pale, listless, and had a mass in the left loin. This had the characteristic of a renal mass in that it moved on respiration and was ballotable. Its nature was confirmed on I.V.P.

540 Nephroblastoma removed at operation from the boy in **539**. Histologically the tumour was composed of tubular and spindle cell components.

541 A transverse section of a nephroblastoma illustrates the variation in consistency often present. It is a greyish to pinkish white colour and is composed of epithelial and connective tissue cells of varying radiosensitivity.

541

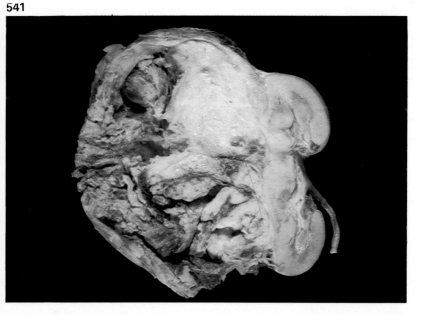

Renal pelvis tumours

542 Papillary carcinoma of the renal pelvis. Tumour is seen at the tip of the instrument. It caused haematuria and was demonstrated on I.V.P. as a space-occupying lesion.

543 Papillary carcinoma The transitional cell tumour of the renal pelvis is similar to that which occurs in the bladder. Haematuria was the presenting symptom.

544 Carcinoma of renal pelvis This more solid tumour of the renal pelvis occurred in a kidney with a double ureter. It was a transitional cell tumour.

542

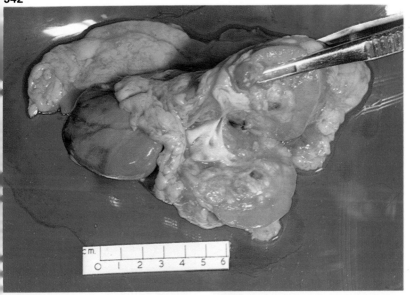

543

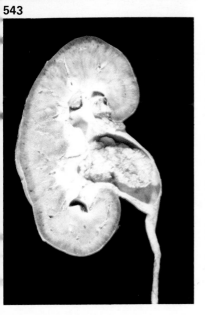

544

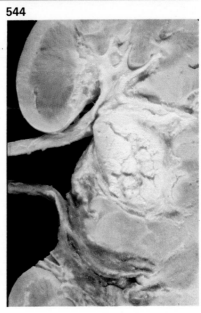

321

Tumours of ureter

These are nearly always malignant. They may be secondary to tumours of renal pelvis or bladder or are primary to the ureter.

Clinical features Haematuria is common. If obstruction occurs then renal pain may be present.

Diagnosis is made by I.V.P. which will show a space-occupying lesion with perhaps proximal dilatation. If the kidney is nonfunctioning it will be necessary to carry out a retrograde pyelogram.

545 Carcinoma of ureter This pathological specimen shows the tumour in the left ureter causing hydronephrosis and metastasis in liver and bone.

546 Carcinoma of ureter This is part of a ureter removed from a patient with recurrent haematuria. The papillary nature is obvious. Diagnosis was made by I.V.P.

545

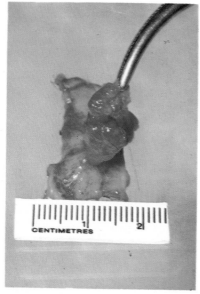

546

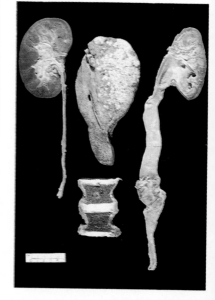

Lesions of the Bladder and Prostate

547 Ectopia vesicae (exstrophy of bladder) The red posterior wall of bladder projects through a defect in the abdominal wall. Fortunately this is not a common congenital condition.

547

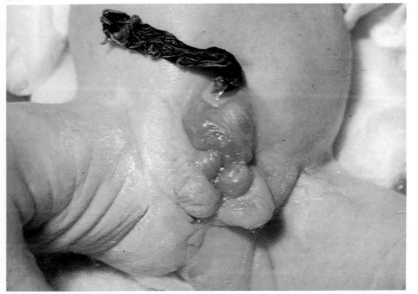

548 Retention of urine produces distension of the bladder which can increase, as here, to above the umbilicus. The patient can be in intense pain if the retention is acute. If chronic it may be almost painless. On examination the bladder is palpated as a tender globular swelling above the pubis. It is dull to percussion and fluctuation can be elicited. An enlarged prostate was felt per rectum.

548

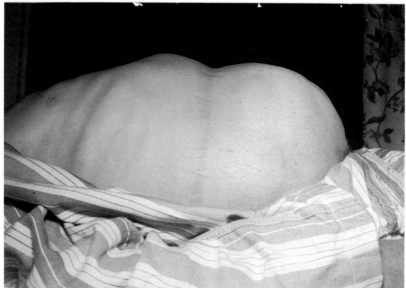

549 Benign hypertrophy of prostate This produces hesitancy at start micturition, a poor slow stream, inadequate emptying, frequency and dribbling at the end. The size of the prostate P.R. is valuable – middle lobe enlargement is not palpable. An I.V.P. and cystogram may show the indentation of the base of the bladder and the residual urine after micturition. Cystoscopy should be done.

549

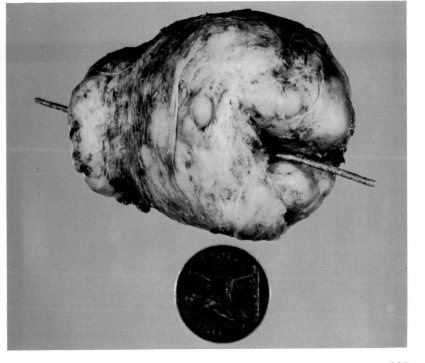

550 Stone in bladder and enlarged prostate The bladder is opened to expose a large mulberry stone resting on an enlarged middle lobe of prostate. This is a calcium oxalate stone coloured due to blood pigment. The symptoms are those of prostatism. Pain is present at the end of micturition or during exercise. It eases off when patient lies down. Haematuria may occur at the end of micturition. Diagnosis is by cystogram and cystoscopy.

551 Stone in bladder This stone formed on a suture which had penetrated the wall of the bladder during repair of a hernia. This emphasises the risk of non-absorbable sutures in operations on the urinary tract.

552 Enlarged prostate and stone This illustrates enlargement of the whole prostate – the middle lobe is prominent. The stones are sometimes called the Jackstone type. The spikes produce pain and haematuria.

550

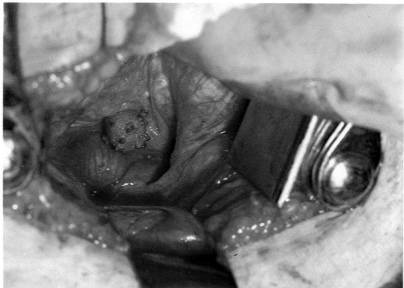

551

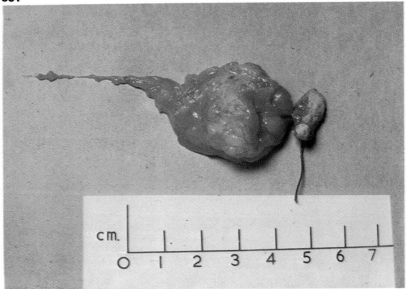

552

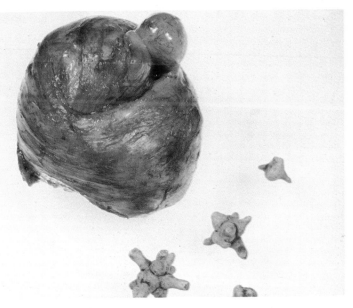

Tumours of the bladder

BENIGN TUMOURS

The most common is the papilloma which in young people is benign but in older age groups should be followed up carefully for recurrence.

MALIGNANT TUMOURS

These are nearly all transitional cell tumours. Rarer types are squamous cell carcinoma, adenocarcinoma and rhabdomyosarcoma.

553 Carcinoma of bladder (transitional cell) usually occurs in the trigonal region but here appears on the side wall of the bladder. The clinical features are haematuria, and symptoms of cystis often present. Diagnosis is based on cystoscopy and biopsy, I.V.P. and cystogram.

554 Cancer of bladder This is a very extensive papillary cancer which infiltrated the vagina to produce a fistula. Symptoms were haematuria, frequency and dysuria.

553

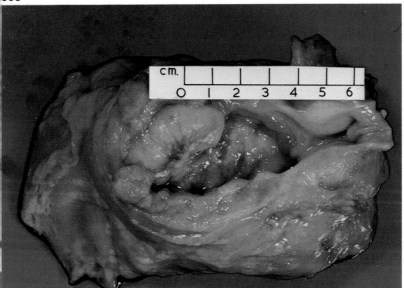

554

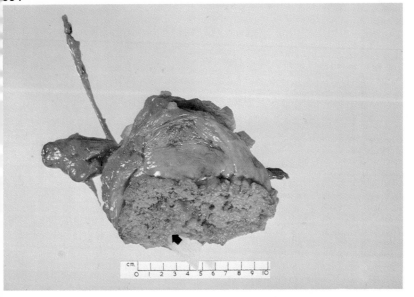

Malignant disease of the prostate

A *carcinoma* nearly always arises in the posterior lobe. Rarely a *sarcoma* may occur.

555 Carcinoma of prostate presents as a cause of bladder neck obstruction. The diagnostic feature is the palpation P.R. of a stony hard nodule or the whole gland may be stony, hard and fixed. A raised acid phosphatase supports the diagnosis, which may be confirmed by biopsy. This patient also had bony metastases and was put on oestrogen, which produced the gynaecomastia.

556 Carcinoma of prostate The secondaries are seen as dense areas in the lumbar spine, sacrum and iliac bones. The patient complained of backache. His acid phosphatase was raised.

555

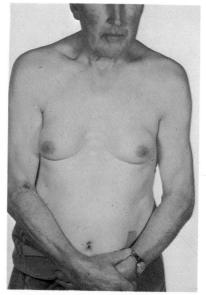

556

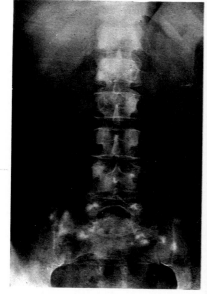

Disease of the Urethra and Penis

557 Urethral valves These may produce obstruction with bilateral hydroureter and hydronephrosis. Diagnosis by urethroscopy and excretory urethrogram.

558 Meatal hypospadias The urethral opening is at the base of the glans. The hooded prepuce comes to the edge of the opening.

557

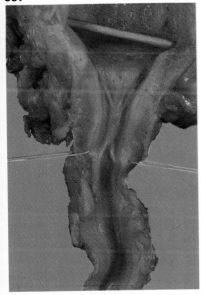

558

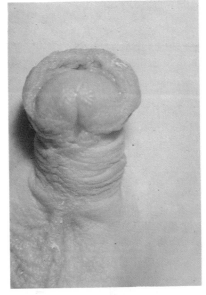

559 Penile hypospadias showing the opening in the midshaft of penis. The hooded prepuce is typical.

560 Perineal hypospadias The scrotum is split and the opening cannot be seen. There is an associated reduplication of the rectum.

561 Meatal stenosis is a congenital narrowing of the end of the urethra. It may be enlarged surgically.

562 Peri-urethral abscess The patient had a stricture of urethra with retention of urine. A suprapubic cystoscopy was done and two weeks later an abscess developed and discharged leaving a shallow ulcer.

563 Rupture of urethra The bruising in the scrotum is visible and the redness above the scrotum spreading outwards to the top of the thigh indicates extravasation of urine.

559

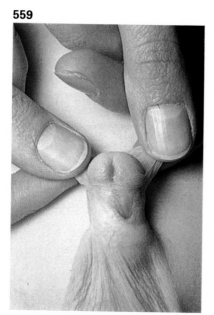

560

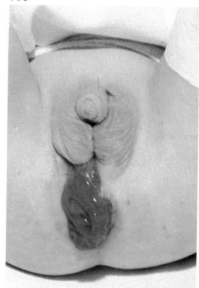

561

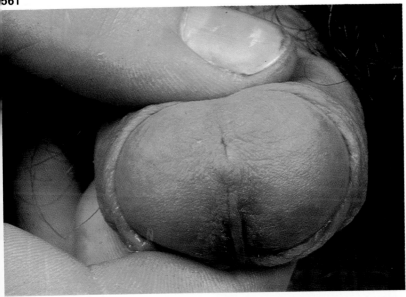

562

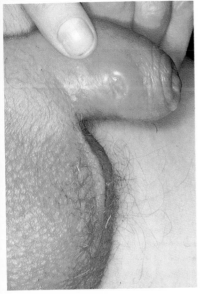

563

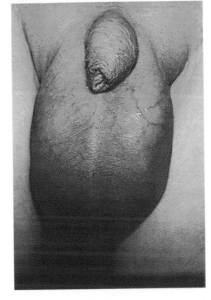

564 Urethrocele (urethral diverticulum) A diverticulum of urethra may occur at an area weakened by injury or rupture of a urethral gland. It is usually found in women. Infection and stone formation may occur. The cystic swelling can be palpated. A bougie passed may be felt to enter the sac. Urethroscopy will demonstrate the opening.

565 Carcinoma of urethra is uncommon. It arises most often in women. The main features are haematuria or bloody spotting of the clothes. Biopsy will confirm the presence of a squamous epithelioma. Tumour nearer to the bladder may be transitional cell cancer.

566 Phimosis is a narrowing of the orifice of the prepuce. It may be congenital, or more often is associated with repeated attacks of balanitis.

567 Oedema of penis The patient had gross oedema of both legs and penis. Lymphoedema was due to blockage of lymphatic glands by secondary tumour.

568 Balanitis is infection of the preputial space. It produces swelling, redness, pain and tenderness of the end of the penis. Pus may be seen exuding in some cases.

564

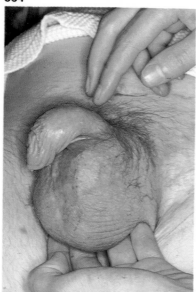

565

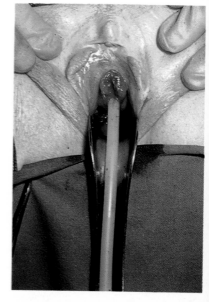

566

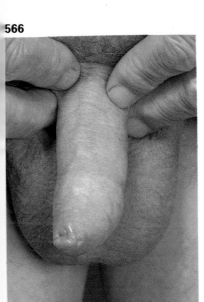

567

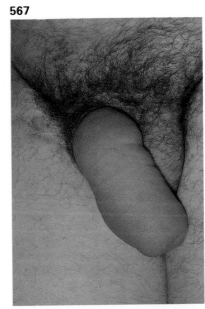

568

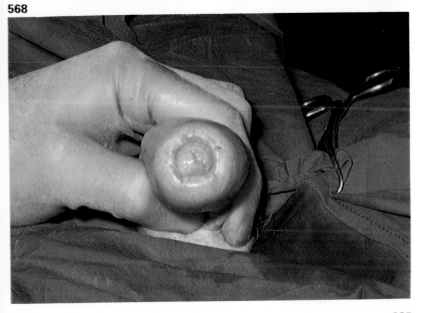

569 Cancer of penis This is a squamous carcinoma which involves the prepuce and glans. The tumour presents as a nodular ulcerative growth. The prepuce may not be retracted and if the tumour lies deep within a dorsal slit may be necessary for diagnosis which differentiates it from a chancre.

570 Cancer of penis The primary growth can be felt but not seen. The enlarged inguinal glands are prominent.

569

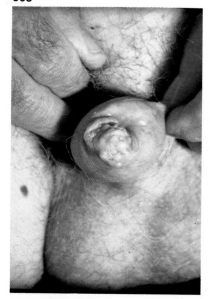

570

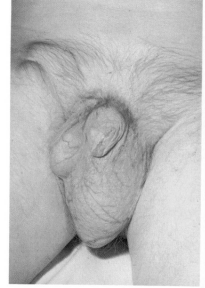

Disease of the Testis, Epididymis and Scrotum

571 An undescended testis is not in the scrotum but lies within the line of descent. In this boy both testes were undescended and lay at the end of the inguinal canal. They could be 'milked' down to the neck of the scrotum. On direct pressure upwards they disappear back into the inguinal canal. The majority descend by puberty.

572 An ectopic testis was present on the right side. It lay outside the line of descent in a pouch above the superficial inguinal ring. Pressure upwards on the testis rendered it more prominent because it could not disappear into the inguinal canal. On the left side the testis could easily be brought down into the scrotum and was therefore a *retractile* testis. If examined in a warm room with warm hands the testis would *lie* in the scrotum.

571

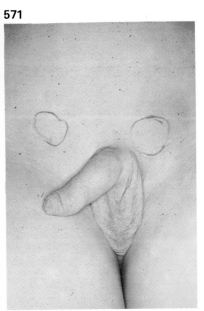

572

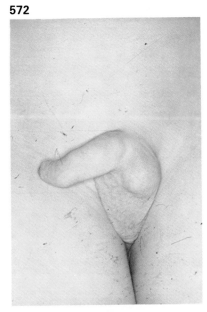

573 Undescended testis The right testis and cord are being mobilised to draw it down into the scrotum. Note poorly developed right side of scrotum. The testis is small.

574 Torsion of the testis The patient complained of sudden onset of lower abdominal pain and tenderness in the scrotum. Redness and tenderness were marked especially on the left side. Although inflammation was considered this is rare in children and torsion was suspected. The cord was felt to be thickened.

575 Torsion of testis At operation the gangrenous left testicle is displayed and the twist in the spermatic cord is evident.

576 Varicocoele is present on the left side of the scrotum. It is a varicosity of the pampiniform plexus which on examination feels like a 'bag of worms'.

573

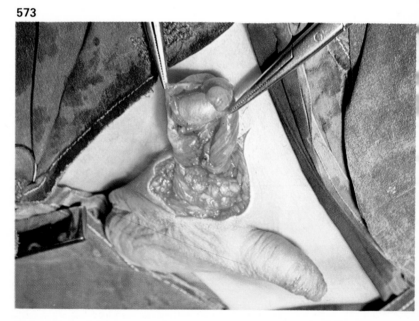

574

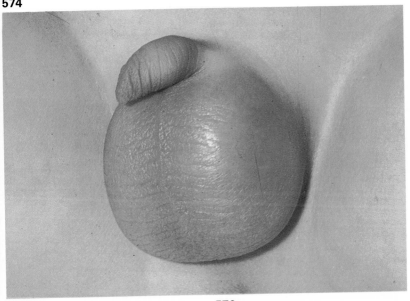

575

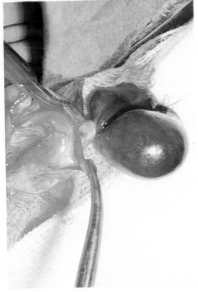

576

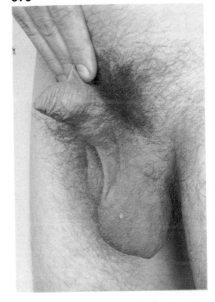

577 Hydrocoele is the accumulation of fluid in the tunica vaginalis. This is shown as a swelling in the left side of the scrotum which has enlarged at the expense of the penis. The testis lies behind the swelling.

578 Hydrocoele The fingers above the swelling denote that it arises in the scrotum and is not an extension from above, i.e. a hernia.

579 Hydrocoele Transillumination shows that the fluid contained is lucent. A small hydrocoele is present on the right side also.

580 Tapped hydrocoele releases a clear, straw-coloured fluid.

581 Hydrocoele of the cord appears as a swelling in the cord above the level of the testis on the right side. It is smooth, cystic and transilluminated.

577

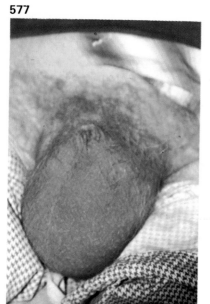

578

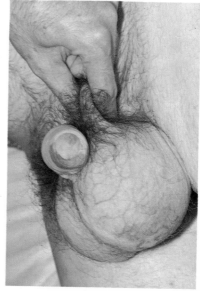

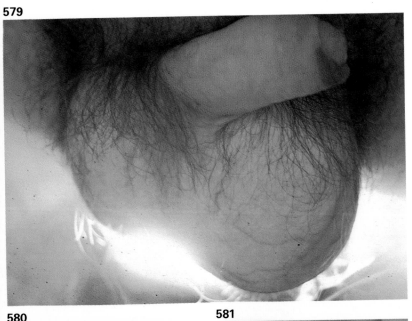

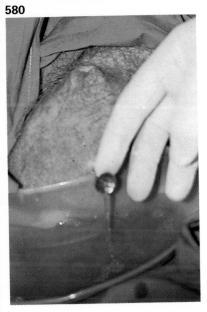

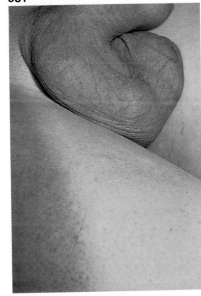

582 A cyst of epididymis also appears as a swelling above the testis but more closely associated. The testis lies below and anterior to the epididymal cyst which does not transilluminate.

583 Epididymitis is present on the right side of the scrotum. The redness and swelling are less intense than that of torsion of the testis. Epididimitis occurs at a later age and may be associated with fever, dysuria, and frequency. Tenderness is most marked posteriorly. The testis itself is not so acutely tender.

584 Tuberculous epididymitis This specimen reveals a thickened nodular epididymis. The condition is not common now. Tenderness and nodularity are posterior to the testis. If it goes on to caseation and sinus formation this will be posterior.

585 Fournier's gangrene of scrotum The clinical features are the sudden appearance of severe inflammation of the whole scrotum. This rapidly progresses on to gangrene affecting also the anterior abdominal wall. It is thought to be the result of a haemolytic streptococcal infection, most probably blood borne.

582

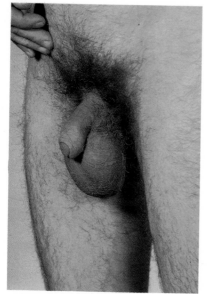

583

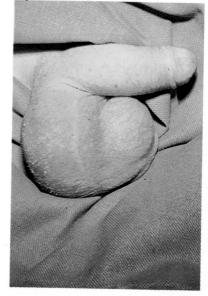

584

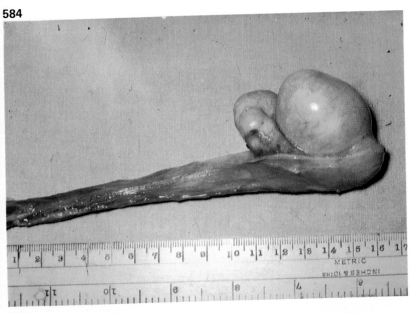

585

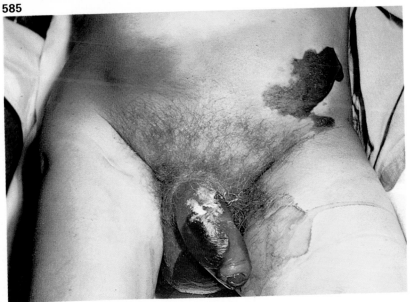

343

Tumours of testis

All tumours of testis are malignant with rare exceptions. They are seen in young men between 18 and 40 years of age.

Clinical features These are a painless swelling firm in consistency in a testis between the ages of 18–40 years. There may be an abdominal mass and gynaecomastia. Tumours can, however, occur in the elderly.

Diagnosis is based on examination, hormonal analysis and x-ray for secondaries and lymphangiography.

586 Seminoma of testis This occurred in a 30-year-old man who noticed the swelling after a bath. It was painless and as it caused no trouble he delayed seeking help for two months. A firm nontender mass was felt in the testis. There was no abdominal mass. Lymphangiography appeared to be normal.

587 Seminoma cut across to show the homogenous appearance of a cream colour.

588 Teratoma of testis arises from toti-potent cells which can form elements from the three layers: ectoderm, mesoderm and endoderm. The tumours on cross-section therefore have a variagated appearance with solid and cystic areas, and, if containing trophoblastic cells, haemorrhagic areas. Depending on the type of cell which prodominates, the teratoma may be classified as embryonal carcinoma, malignant teratoma, chorion carcinoma.

589 Gynaecomastia in a young man of 30 years should raise the suspicion of a tumour of testis. He had a mass in the left testis which was a chorion carcinoma.

586

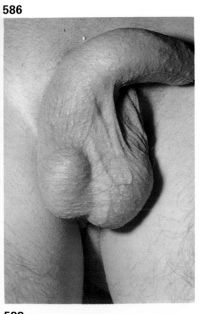

587

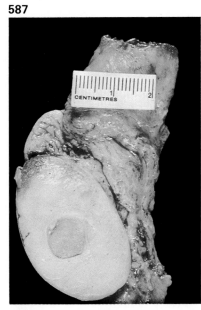

588

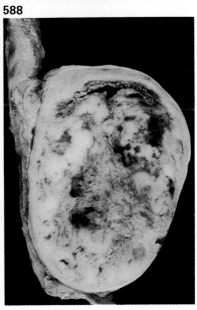

589

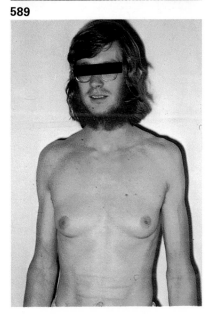

345

590 Lymphosarcoma of the testis seen in an elderly patient. The tumour was nodular and extended upwards to the external ring on the left side. It is debateable as to whether this tumour is primary in the testis or part of a lymphosarcoma elsewhere. No other lesion was found.

591 Lymphosarcoma of testis The cut section of the lesion mentioned in **590** is shown. It has a variagated appearance suggestive of teratoma but the histology was that of lymphosarcoma.

592 Carcinoma of epididymis There was a hard swelling in the right side of the scrotum. The testis lay in front of the mass which extended above. It was obviously arising from the epididymis. As tumours of the epididymis are rare the possibility of a chronic epididymitis was considered.

593 Carcinoma of epididymis The tumour is seen almost surrounding the testis. This emphasises the point that not all swellings of the epididymis are inflammatory.

590

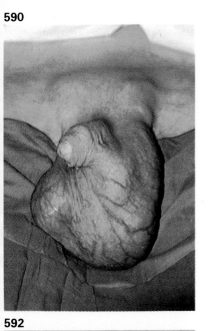

591

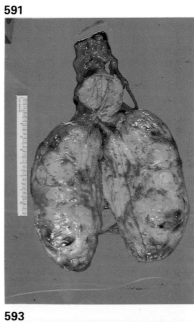

592

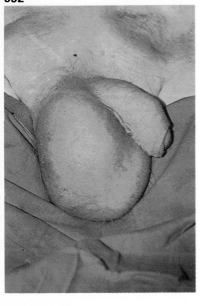

593

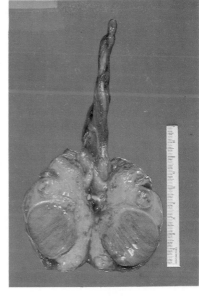

Disease of Thyroid and Parathyroid

Chronic thyroiditis

This curious condition occurs in three forms: *Hashimoto's disease, granulomatous thyroiditis* and *Reidel's thyroiditis.*

595 Hashimoto's disease It is not always easy to exclude cancer in all cases. Total thyroidectomy was carried out here. The cut surface shows the large nodules which may produce a bosselated surface on examination. The colour is pale pink to yellow. History shows replacement of thyroid tissue by lymphoid follicles. Auto antibody titres in the blood would have helped in diagnosis.

596 Riedel's thyroiditis is rare and is recognisable by touch. The thyroid feels like a hard woody mass due to marked fibrosis. Infiltration of the surroundings by the fibrosis makes one think of cancer. Biopsy with frozen section is necessary for diagnosis.

Thyroid deficiency

596 Myxoedema is characterised by a gradually increasing lethargy, mental and physical. The face becomes coarser. The hair is prematurely grey, dry and falls out. Thinning of the lateral margins of the eyebrows may be noticeable. Diagnosis will be confirmed by elevated serum cholesterol and low protein-bound iodine.

594

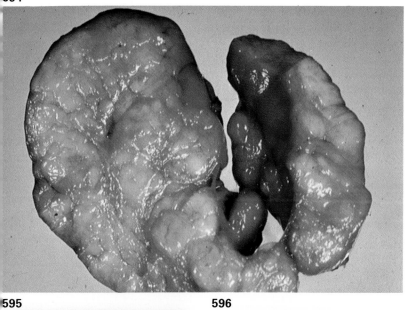

595

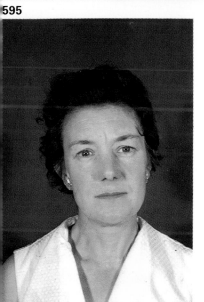

596

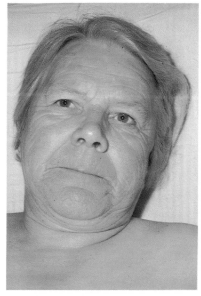

Goitre

597 Nontoxic diffuse (simple) goitre This may be physiological
(puberty, pregnancy, menopause), endemic, or result of goitrogenic agents.
The swelling of the thyroid may grow to large size producing dyspnoea or
dysphagia. The surface is smooth and soft to firm consistency.

598 Colloid goitre is seen in periods of psychological stress. The whole
gland is enlarged and may bulge outwards markedly. The swelling is smooth
and has an elastic feel.

599 A nodular goitre is associated with iodine deficiency. The thyroid is
enlarged asymmetrically and the surface is firm and nodular. One of the
nodules may be large enough to suggest a neoplasm. Cystic change is
evident.

597

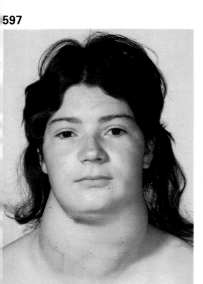

598

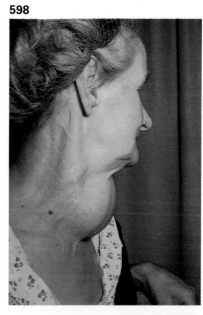

599

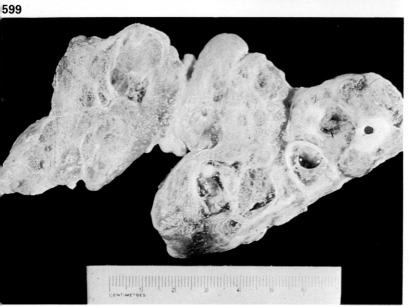

600 Retro-tracheal thyroid Thyroid enlargement may occur outwards as in **598**, downwards into the retrosternal area, and backwards to press on the trachea or as in this case to pass behind and surround the trachea.

601 Primary toxic goitre The thyroid gland is uniformly enlarged, feels firm and smooth, and a thyroid thrill or bruit may be present. The symptoms are nervousness, irritability, sweating, increased appetite but loss of weight, intolerance to heat, a warm moist skin, tachycardia and hand tremors.

602 Thyrotoxicosis may arise as a diffuse goitre (*Grave's disease*) or from a nodular goitre, or a toxic adenoma. A prominent sign is exophthalmos which occurs especially in the primary toxic goitre. The sclera is visible all round the cornea giving the typical startled look.

603 Primary toxic goitre The specimen obtained by subtotal thyroidectomy gives some idea of the increased vascularity. The hyperfunction results in an elevated P.B.I., increased radioiodine uptake and radio-T_3 uptake.

600

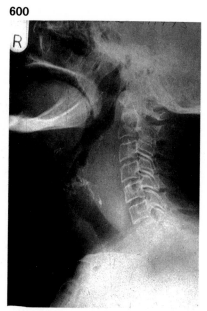

601

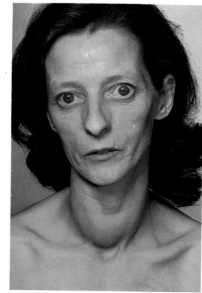

602

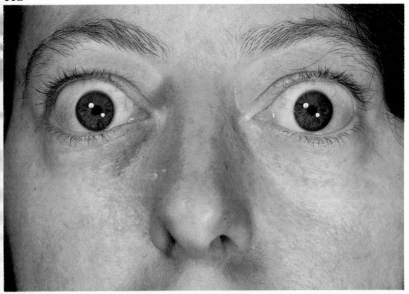

603

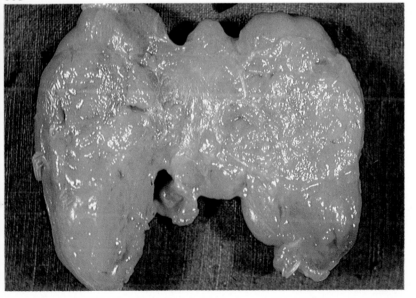

604 Secondary thyrotoxicosis occurs in a pre-existing goitre or adenoma. Cardiovascular symptoms tend to predominate and may lead to cardiac failure and diabetes as in this patient.

605 Pretibral oedema is an uncommon sign in thyrotoxicosis and is seen in this patient with marked cardiovascular symptoms.

606 Progressive exophthalmos is a distressing but fortunately rare condition. Despite ablation of the thyroid the condition progresses with proptosis, deterioration of vision, corneal ulceration, chemosis, papilloedema and finally, if not averted, an ophthalmoplegia and panophthalmitis (*malignant exophthalmos*).

607 Adenoma of thyroid is seen in this resected specimen as a large mass at one pole of the thyroid. It was easily felt clinically as a solitary swelling which moved on swallowing. It is best excised as it could be malignant at the outset, or become so.

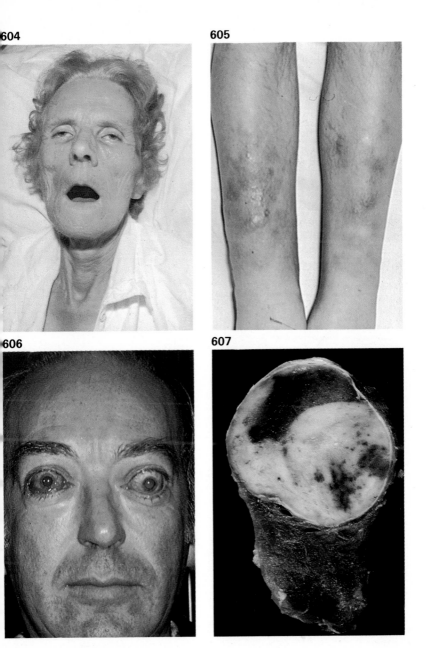

604

605

606

607

355

Malignant tumours of the thyroid

Malignant tumours of the thyroid are classified as: *papillary adenocarcinoma* – 60%, *follicular adenocarcinoma* – 20%, *undifferentiated carcinoma* – 15%, *medullary carcinoma* – 5%.

608 Papillary adenocarcinoma is a slow growing tumour of childhood or early adult life. This patient had a swelling of the left lobe of thyroid for four years and finally came up with the enlarged glands in the neck.

608

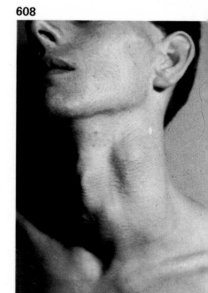

609 Papillary adenocarcinoma of thyroid A total thyroidectomy was carried out in the patient in **608** with removal of glands in the neck.

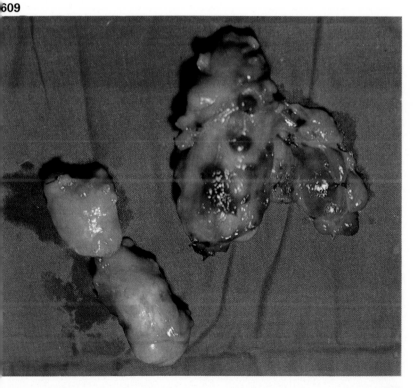

610 Undifferentiated carcinoma of the thyroid is a rapidly growing tumour of middle age and later. It is more common in women. This man noticed a thickening of his neck with a need for a larger neck size in his shirt. Swallowing was uncomfortable and his voice had become hoarse. On examination both lobes of the thyroid were enlarged, the right more so than the left. The gland was fixed.

611 Medullary cancer of the thyroid presents as a solitary hard nodule of the thyroid. The specimen shows the nodule in the upper pole and the spread to lymphatic glands. Diarrhoea may be a prominant feature.

610

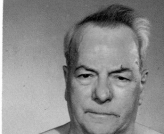

611

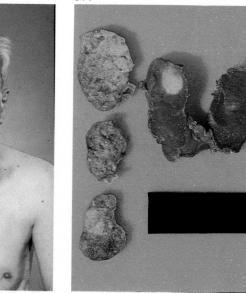

Parathyroid

612 Hyperparathyroidism is usually due to a single adenoma as shown here. Other causes are multiple adenomas, hyperplasia, and rarely, carcinoma. The diagnosis rests on a raised serum calcium (> 11 mg/100 ml), a para normal serum phosphate, and changes in the bones.

613 Hyperparathyroidism The simultaneous occurrence of gallstones and renal stones should intensify investigations to exclude the presence of parathyroidism.

612

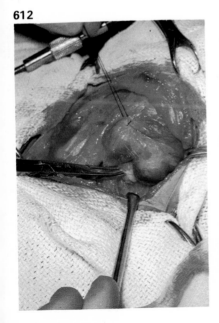

613

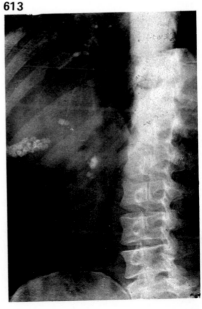

614 Hyperparathyroidism The typical radiological picture is a subperiosteal resorption of bone best seen in the middle phalanges. Other changes
are a resorption of the tufts of the fingers and a homogeneous ground glass
pattern of the calvarium.

614

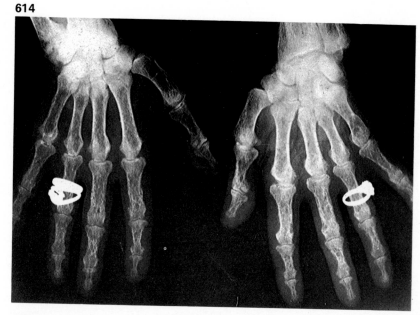

Disease of the Thymus and Adrenal

Thymus

615 An adenoma of thymus is a benign tumour. This one was removed from a patient with myasthenia gravis. There followed a marked improvement in her condition with the need for much less neostigmine.

616 A thymoma is the malignant tumour of the thymus. It is highly malignant and produces clinical features by compression of the tracheal and the vessels in the superior mediastinum. The illustration shows a recurrence of a thymoma sometime after the surgical extirpation.

615

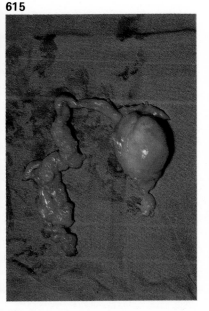

616

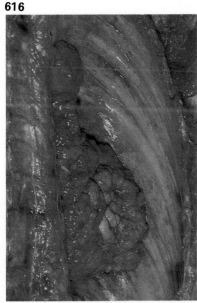

Adrenal

Disease of the adrenal affects the cortex or medulla or both. It may result in the secretion of excessive amounts of hormones producing characteristic syndrome.

LESIONS OF THE ADRENAL CORTEX

These types of lesions are bilateral hyperplasia, benign adenoma, and carcinoma. The clinical features depend on the hormone released in excess.

617 Aldosteronism This is classified as primary aldosteronism *(Conn's syndrome)* if due to a cortical adenoma, and secondary aldosteronism if secondary to disease of the cardiovascular system or kidneys. The illustration is a cortical adenoma found in a patient with the features of primary aldosteronism; hypertension due to retention of sodium, muscular weakness due to hypokalaemia and alkalosis. Diagnosis can be confirmed by a low plasma renin level and a high urinary aldosterone level.

617

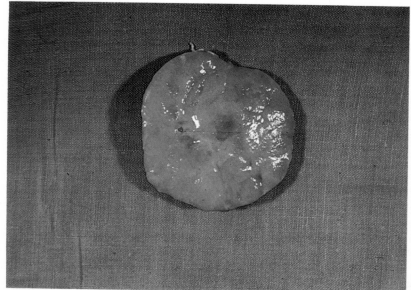

618 Cushing's syndrome is due to hypersecretion of cortisol and corticosterone. The clinical features are: moon face, buffalo type obesity, striae, amenorrhoea, hirsuitism, hypertension, glycosuria and osteoporosis. Hypokalaemia and hypochloraemia are present with a raised 17-hydroxycorticosteroid level. Radiology may demonstrate enlargement of the adrenals, one or both. A pituitary tumour should be excluded.

619 The cortical adenoma excised from the patient in **618**.

618

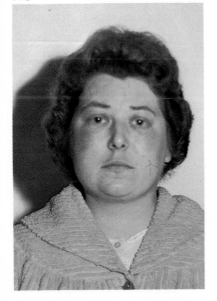

619

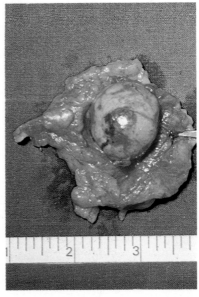

620 Cushing's syndrome (post operation) Excision of the adenoma resulted in a disappearance of the features illustrated in **618**.

621 Cushing's syndrome illustrating the hirsuitism and buffalo type obesity. This man noticed that he bruised easily and was impotent.

622 A hyperplastic adrenal gland found in a patient with Cushing's disease.

620

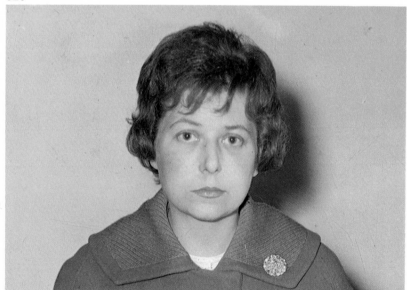

621

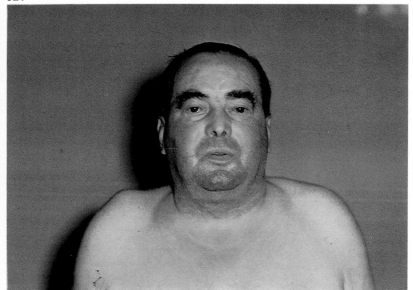

622

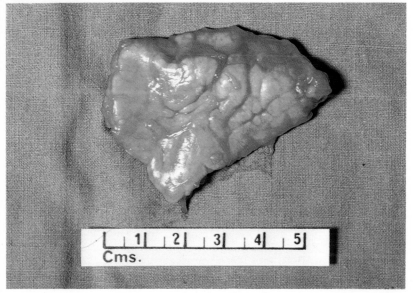

623 Cushing's syndrome in the young and the elderly is sometimes due to carcinoma of the adrenal. This carcinoma was removed from a 70-year-old patient with a short history. The level of urinary 17-oxogenic steroids was over 100 mg; a diagnostic feature of carcinoma. The angiogram showed the presence of a vascular tumour of the right adrenal.

624 Adrenogenital syndrome is due to excessive production of androgens from hyperplasia or tumour. In this 7-year-old boy it produced a precocious puberty. In females it would cause virilism. The 17-oxosteroids level in the urine was high. Retroperitoneal insufflation showed the presence of a tumour.

623

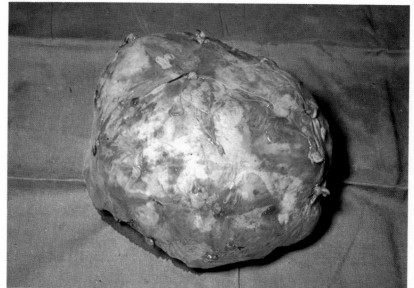

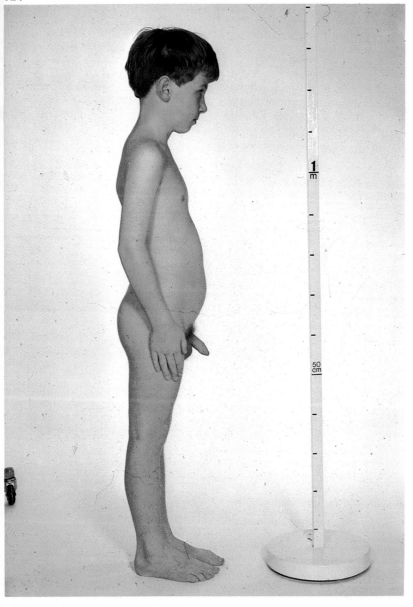

LESIONS OF ADRENAL MEDULLA

625 A phaeochromocytoma is a tumour of adrenal medulla which releases excess adrenaline or noradrenaline (or both). The clinical features depend on the relative proportions of these hormones. The patient may have attacks of headaches, vasomotor changes, visual disturbances, sweating and pallor due to paroxysmal hypertension. In others sustained hypertension may be present. The urinary catecholamines or their metabolites vanillyl mandelic acid (V.M.A.) will be raised. The tumour is a homogenous brown colour.

626 A ganglioneuroma is usually a symptomless benign tumour presenting as a mass. It can however also secrete excess of catecholamines, and may produce hypertension.

627 A neuroblastoma is a highly malignant tumour of the sympathetic neurones in the adrenal medulla. It is usually seen in infants as an enlarging mass in the loin rather like a Wilm's tumour. I.V.P. will help to differentiate the two.

625

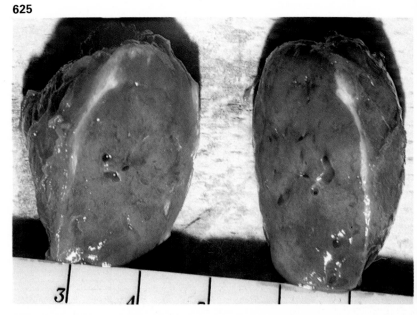

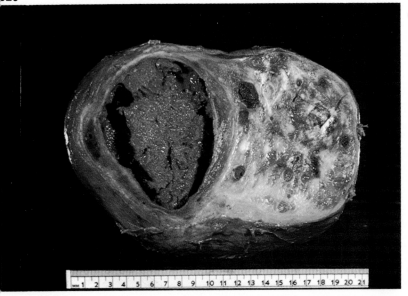

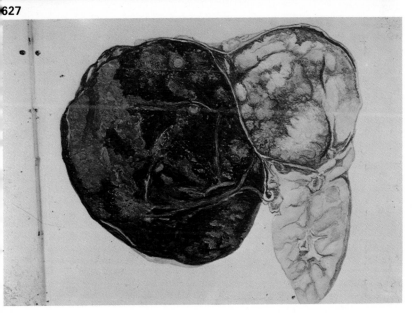

ADRENAL FAILURE

This may be acute as in the adrenal apoplexy in the newborn, the Waterhouse-Friderichsen syndrome, or following surgery in a patient previously on steroid therapy. Chronic failure is seen in Addison's disease.

628 Waterhouse-Friderichsen syndrome is seen as a complication of septicaemia especially of the fulminant meningococoel variety. The features are of sudden collapse with vomiting, hyperpyrexia, cyanosis, and petechial haemorrhages into the skin. These coalesce into purpuric blotches. Diagnosis is usually made from clinical features and response to the intravenous hydrocortisone.

629 Addison's disease A characteristic feature of this chronic insufficiency of the adrenal cortex is the dusky pigmentation of the skin seen here in the face. It also occurs at points of pressure, i.e. on the abdominal wall.

630 Pigmentation of the hard palate was the only sign of Addison's disease in a patient who collapsed after an operation and was resuscitated by hydrocortisone. Later tests of water excretion and the low urinary 17-keto-steroids supported the diagnosis.

628

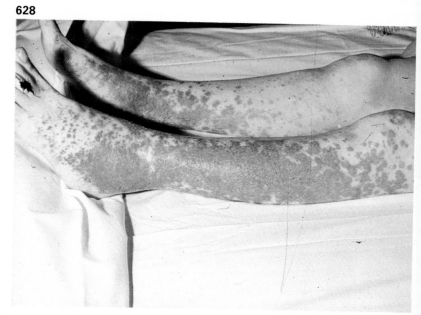

629

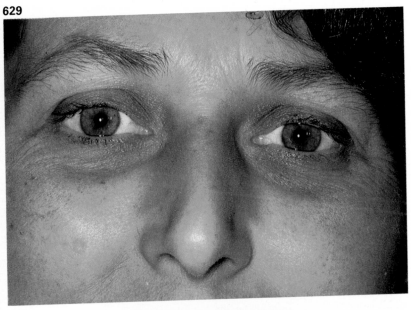

630

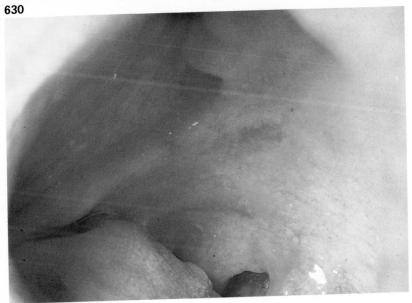

631 Pigmentation of the skin of a patient with Addison's disease is compared with a normal individual.

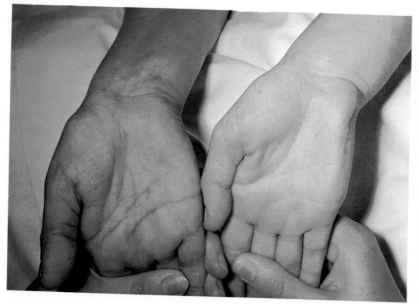

Hernia

Classification of anatomical varieties

Diaphragmatic – congenital, traumatic, incisional

Oesophageal (hiatus) – sliding, paraoesophageal (rolling), mixed

Umbilical – congenital, adult

Inguinal – indirect, direct, interstitial

Femoral

Incisional

Epigastric

Rare types – obturator, sciatic, vaginal, lumbar, pudendal, prevascular, femoral, and intra-abdominal herniae in relation to peritoneal folds

632 Congenital diaphragmatic hernia presents as an extreme emergency in a new born baby who is cyanosed and breathless due to presence of part of the gut in the chest (nearly always on the left side). In this 3-hour-old child part of the liver, stomach and small bowel are present in the chest.

633 Congenital diaphragmatic hernia A barium meal shows the left chest filled with small bowel. The left lung is completely collapsed.

632

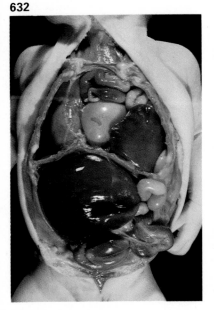

633

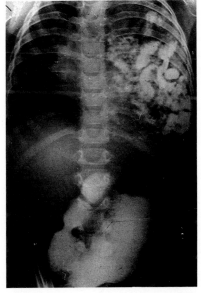

634 Congenital umbilical hernia usually appears as a small skin covered swelling at the umbilicus which is prominent when the child strains, and is easily reducible. This is an example of the severest type of umbilical hernia, the omphalocoele.

635 Adult para-umbilical hernia This is a swelling in the area of the umbilicus. Here it is small, but it may be quite large. It is usually irreducible and may strangulate with pain, tenderness and vomiting.

636 Indirect right inguinal hernia The hernial contents pass through the deep inguinal ring, out the external ring and down towards the scrotum. It passes medial to the pubic tubercle. On lying down the hernia may reduce itself or be easily pushed back.

637 The congenital inguinal hernia passing down into the tunica vaginalis is seen in young children and may quickly become strangulated.

634

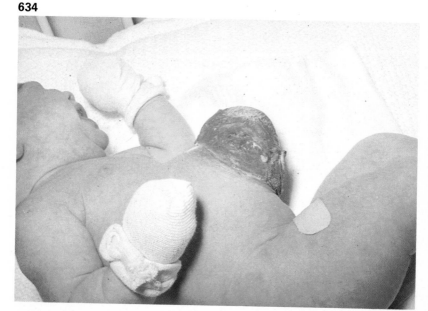

635

636

637

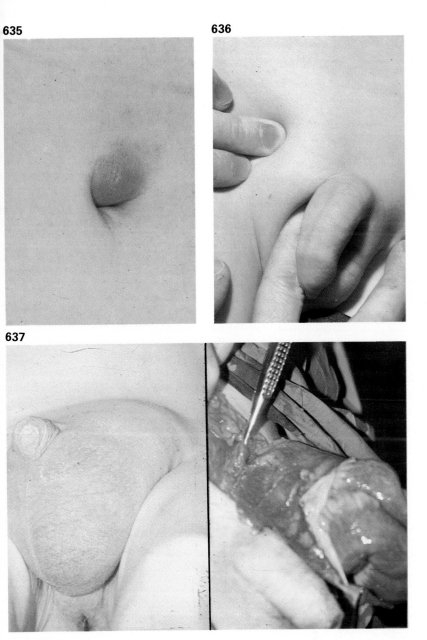

375

638 Direct inguinal hernia passes directly through the external inguinal ring. It does not enter the scrotum. On reduction a gap will be felt in the conjoint tendon. It is seen most commonly in elderly males. It is shown here on the right side with an indirect hernia on the left side.

639 The same hernia is reduced directly backwards. The finger is shown passing through the external ring and the gap in the conjoint tendon.

640 The femoral hernia passes behind the inguinal ligament down into the thigh via the femoral canal. It is thus lateral to and below the pubic tubercle.

641 Femoral hernia This demonstrates the relationship to the tubercle which can be detected by abducting the thigh and passing the finger up along the adductor longus muscle.

638

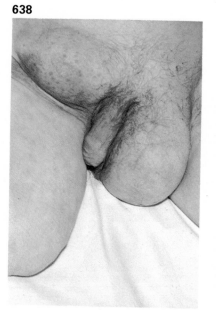

639

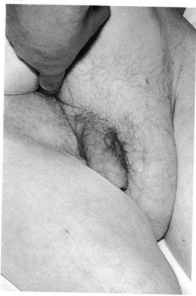

640

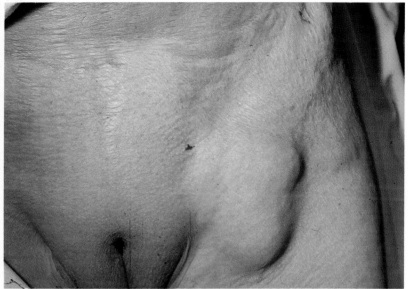

641

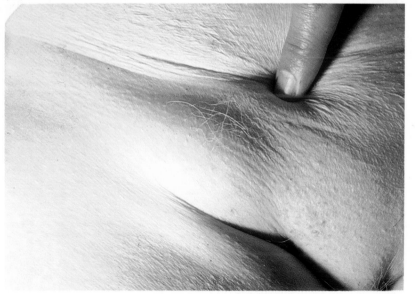

377

642 Femoral hernia may be so small as to be difficult to feel, or as in this case, very large.

643 Femoral hernia This patient complained of a painful tender swelling in the right groin. It was defined as a femoral hernia complete with sac.

644 Femoral hernia – strangulated The congested segment of the circumference of the small bowel loculated in the hernia is the Richter hernia. This is dangerous as it does not produce obstructive symptoms and can easily be missed.

645 An incisional hernia occurs through any scar in the abdomen. Midline lower abdominal scars are notorious for giving way. In this case the hernia is through a colostomy incision.

646 A large ventral incisional hernia is seen occasionally. It causes great discomfort to the patient and is usually irreducible. Operative reduction of such a hernia could seriously embarrass respiration.

642

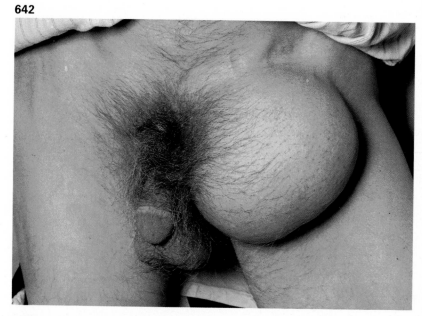

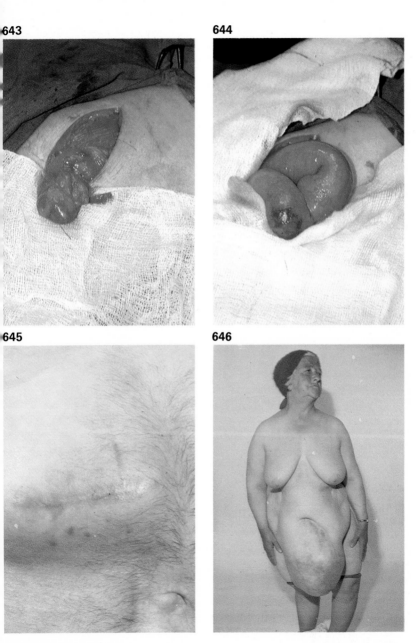

643

644

645

646

647 A large incisional hernia containing small bowel incarcerated in the hernia. Intestinal obstruction was present.

648 Strangulation of an incisional hernia is signified by central abdominal pain due to intestinal obstruction, pain and tenderness in the region of the swelling and redness of the overlying skin.

649 At operation the strangulated loop of small bowel is seen. The damage was irreversible and the bowel had to be resected with end to end anastomosis.

650 An epigastric hernia is usually a small protrusion of extraperitoneal fat through the linea alba. It normally requires no treatment but occasionally the fat may be traumatised and become painful. The hernia is shown being dissected out.

647

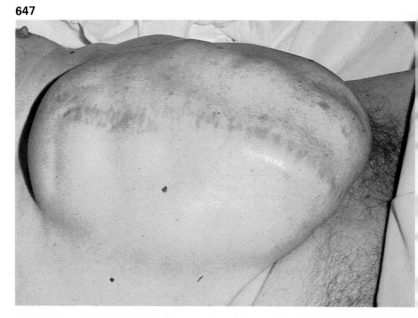

648

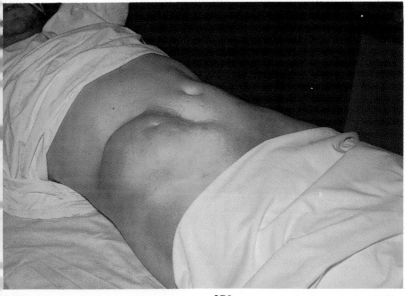

649

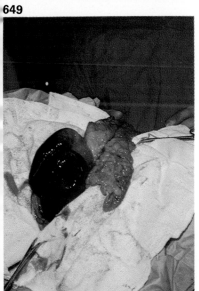

650

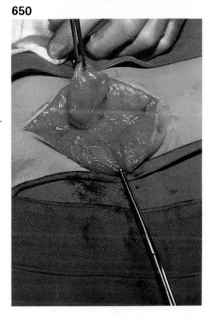

651 A perineal hernia is one of the rare types where the protrusion has occurred through the muscles of the pelvic floor. This may cause difficulty in sitting, or urinary problems.

651

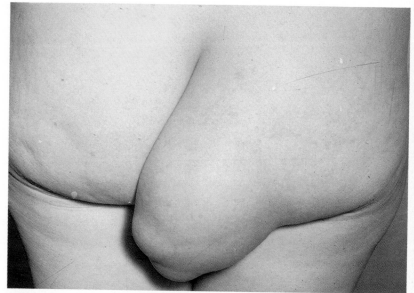

Arterial Disease

652 General clinical features of arterial disease are related to the vessel affected and the degree of ischaemia produced.

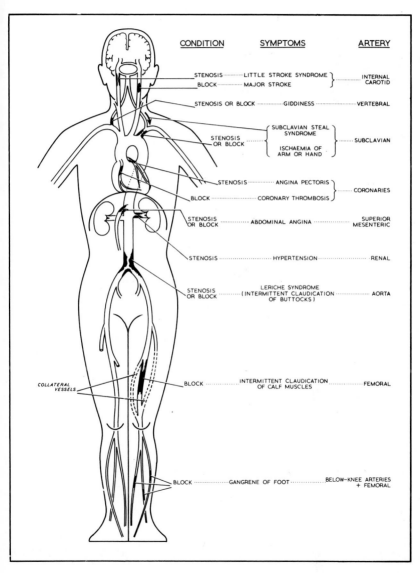

CONDITION	SYMPTOMS	ARTERY
STENOSIS	LITTLE STROKE SYNDROME	INTERNAL CAROTID
BLOCK	MAJOR STROKE	
STENOSIS OR BLOCK	GIDDINESS	VERTEBRAL
STENOSIS OR BLOCK	SUBCLAVIAN STEAL SYNDROME / ISCHAEMIA OF ARM OR HAND	SUBCLAVIAN
STENOSIS	ANGINA PECTORIS	CORONARIES
BLOCK	CORONARY THROMBOSIS	
STENOSIS OR BLOCK	ABDOMINAL ANGINA	SUPERIOR MESENTERIC
STENOSIS	HYPERTENSION	RENAL
STENOSIS OR BLOCK	LERICHE SYNDROME (INTERMITTENT CLAUDICATION OF BUTTOCKS)	AORTA
BLOCK	INTERMITTENT CLAUDICATION OF CALF MUSCLES	FEMORAL
BLOCK	GANGRENE OF FOOT	BELOW-KNEE ARTERIES + FEMORAL

COLLATERAL VESSELS

653 Rubor on dependency is a sign of a diminished vis a tergo due to arterial blockage. The blood is thus returned from the feet against gravity only with difficulty.

654 Pallor on elevation When both legs are lifted and blood has to be pushed up against the force of gravity the ischaemic foot will become pale. The pallor is seen on the toes and distal foot. The same effect can be produced by making the patient paddle his feet in this position until claudication is experienced. Again the foot of the affected limb will become pale.

655 Atheromatous material shown in a common site, the abdominal aorta. The atheroma has ulcerated in places and has produced damage to the renal arteries.

656 Femoral artery block The atheromatous plug excised from the femoral artery is shown. This artery has a vein patch inserted to keep the lumen open. The patient complained of pain in the calf on walking a 100 yards (intermittent claudication). The femoral artery pulse could be felt but none distally.

653

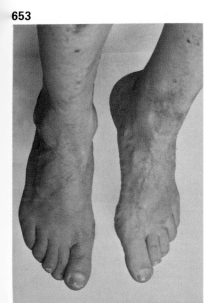

654

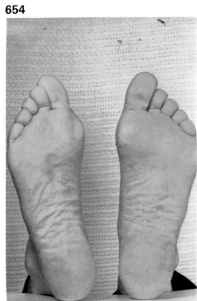

655

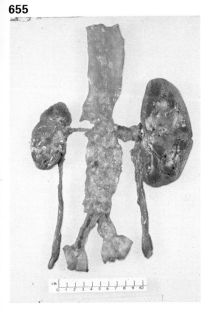

656

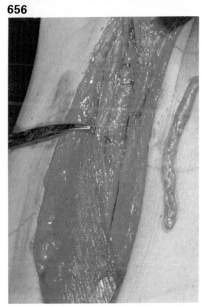

657 Femoral artery block The diagnosis and exact site of blockage are confirmed by an arteriogram. The femoral artery should be seen passing from the mid-inguinal region to cross the femur at the junction of the middle and lower third. The profunda femoris artery is present and crosses the bone at the junction of the middle and upper third.

658 Thermography is a new technique which measures the infra red emission from the limb. Hot areas with good blood flow are white, and cold ischaemic areas black. In a femoral block there is characteristically a warm area round the block and the knee due to collateral flow and a cold area distally.

659 The femoral pulse is easily felt below the mid-point of the inguinal ligament. The pulses on either side should be compared. Weakness on one side or a bruit on auscultation would suggest more proximal stenosis.

660 The popliteal pulse is usually felt with the knee bent and muscles relaxed. The finger of the examining hand palpates the popliteal fossa with the thumb just above the tibial tuberosity. One hand overlies the other to give further compression in a difficult case. The pulse is not always easily felt even when present.

657

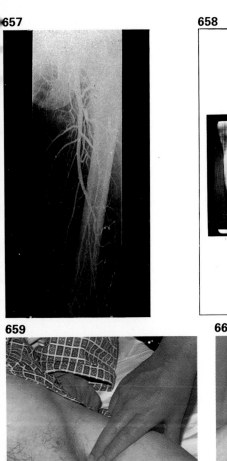

658

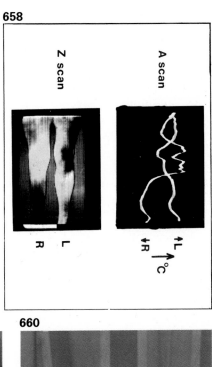

Z scan

A scan

L
R

↑L
↓R
→°C

659

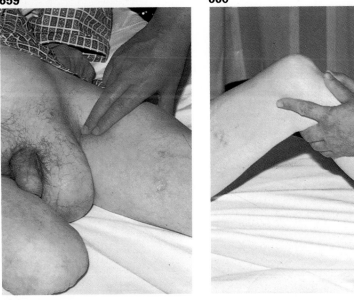

660

387

661 The posterior tibial pulse is felt in the groove midway between the medial condyle and the heel. If present it is usually reasonably easy to feel.

662 The dorsalis pedis pulse is felt on the dorsum of the foot just lateral to the tendon of the extensor hallucis muscle. This also is normally an easy pulse to feel.

663 Blockage of the arteries below the knee shown in this arteriogram may produce severe ischaemia of the foot with rest pain. This pain is felt in the forefoot especially during the night and is of a burning character although the foot feels cold to touch. It is relieved by putting the foot out of bed and especially on a cold floor.

664 A typical dry gangrene of the big toe seen in an elderly man with a block in the femoral artery and blockage of the vessels below the knee with poor collateral circulation.

665 Moist gangrene occurs in tissues containing excess fluid. The example shown is gangrene in a diabetic where infection was prominent. Moist gangrene also occurs in venous blockage.

661

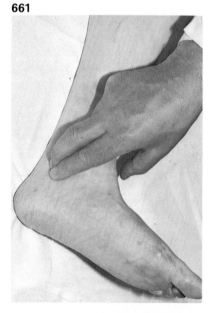

662

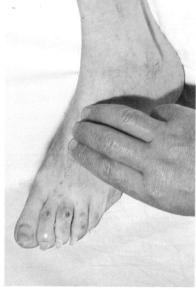

663

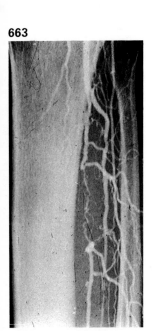

664

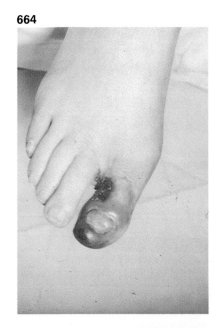

665

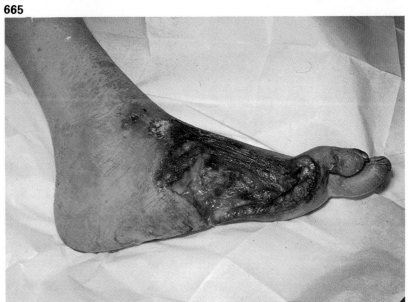

666 An arteriogram of a patient with severe ischaemia of the right leg and claudication in other side. The atheromatous material removed from the lower aorta is shown alongside it. The plug from the right common iliac artery narrowing is superimposed on the narrowed area.

667 Carotid artery stenosis shown on this arteriogram as a marked narrowing. This produces the typical syndrome of recurrent episodes of weakness of one side of the body present for a few minutes – small stroke syndrome. Visual disturbances may be present. On auscultation a bruit may be heard over the carotid bifurcation and a thrill may be felt.

668 The internal carotid artery has been opened with an extension into the common carotid. The atheromatous material is visible and the silk tie leads down to an internal shunt to allow blood flow to continue while the atheroma is being excised.

669 Narrowing of the subclavian artery shown here on the left side can lead to a reverse in blood flow in the left vertebral artery when the left hand is exercised. This can produce dizziness and even blackout – the *subclavian steal syndrome.* On the right the plug removed from the artery is superimposed on the narrowed area.

666

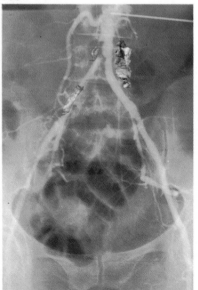

667

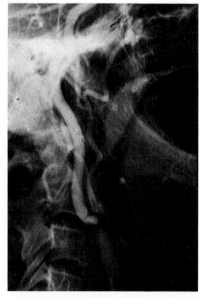

668

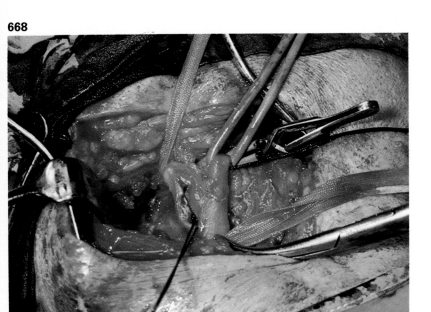

669

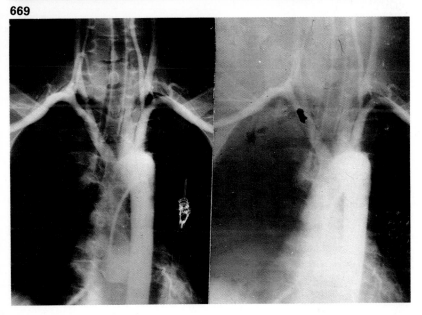

670 Narrowing of the renal artery may produce hypertension and on auscultation a bruit may be audible on one or even both sides of the midline in the epigastrium. Diagnostic investigations include split renal function tests, renin estimations and renal blood flow. Arteriography delineates the site of blockage.

671 Narrowing of the renal artery may be relieved by excision and anastomosis or by a dacron graft from aorta to renal artery beyond the point of narrowing as shown here. Following this the blood pressure fell to near normal.

672 Ischaemia of the alimentary canal may be sudden and catastrophic with gangrene of the bowel or chronic due to occlusion of the coeliac axis. This may be due to atheromatous narrowing of the coeliac, and either the superior or inferior mesenteric arteries or to compression of the coeliac axis by a band. The coeliac axis is shown dissected out.

673 The scissors lie in front of the coeliac axis and demonstrate the compression band which was incised.

670

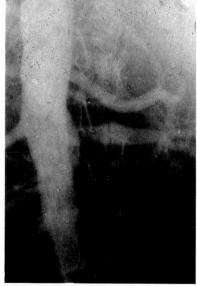

671

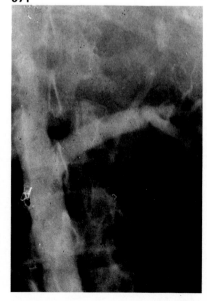

672

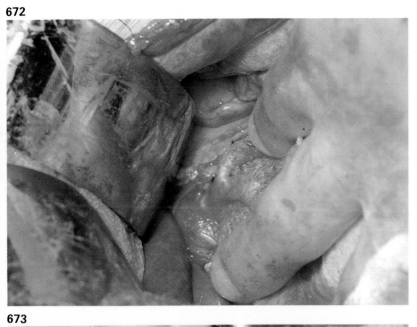

673

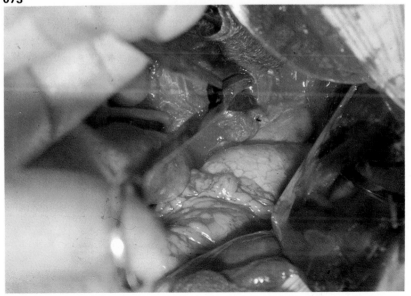

674 Abdominal aortic aneurysms are nearly all due to atherosclerosis. The aneurysm may cause a throbbing discomfort in the abdomen with pain in the back. The swelling can be palpated and exhibits expansile palpation. Arteriography is usually not necessary to establish the diagnosis. The tape surrounds the lower end of the aorta at its bifurcation.

675 The whole abdominal aneurysm is shown excised in this case with the bifurcation. A trouser graft of dacron is used to restore continuity. These aneurysms can grow quite large and may rupture causing acute abdominal and back pain and collapse.

676 A popliteal aneurysm The old man complained of a throbbing pain behind the knee. The pain had become more persistent before admission and his foot was cold. One noticed the bruising behind the knee and a tender pulsating mass.

677 An arteriogram can demonstrate the popliteal aneurysm in a patient presenting with a swelling behind the knee.

674

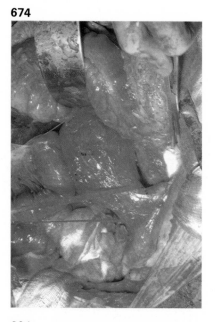

675

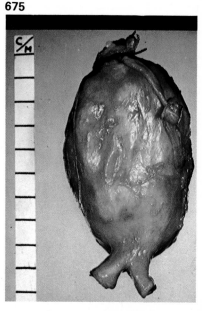

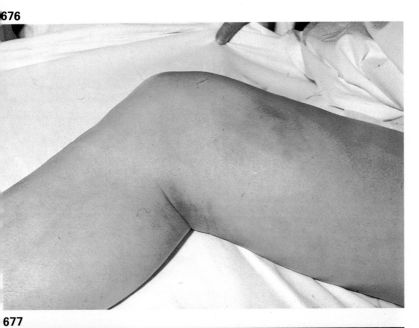

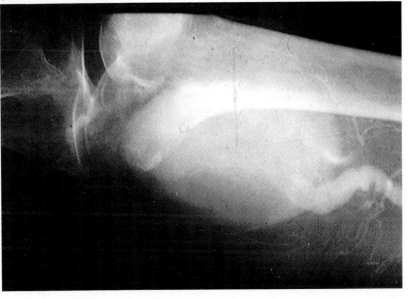

678 A dissection of the popliteal fossa of the same patient who died suddenly before operation could be performed. The atheromatous artery, the blood clot, and the leak into surrounding tissues are evident.

679 Acute arterial occlusion may be due to embolism, thrombosis, or trauma. The skin is at first pale then a mottled cyanosis appears. Anaesthesia and loss of function develop and pulses distal to the site of blockage are absent. If unilateral gangrene may develop.

680 An embolus is characterised by sudden onset of coldness, numbness and pain in the limb. It is removed as here, by a Fogarty catheter which is inserted and a balloon at the end blown up. As the catheter is withdrawn the balloon pulls out the clot. The pale embolus is seen with fresh thrombus adjacent.

678

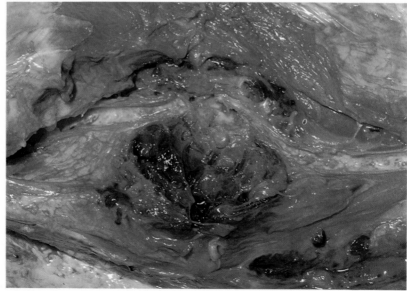

679

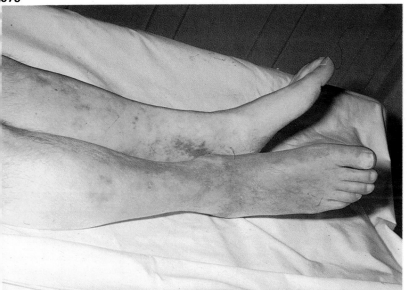

680

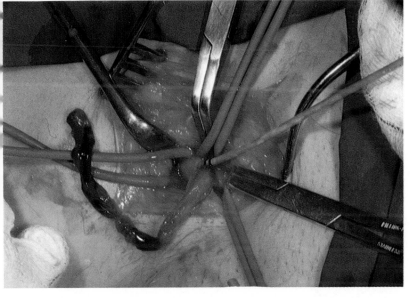

681 Thromboangitis obliterans (Buerger's disease) affects the small arteries of the hands or feet producing occlusions and is frequently accompanied by migratory phlebitis. It occurs in young cigarette smoking males. Digital ischaemia progresses to gangrene and amputation. This patient was unusual in being a female.

682 Raynaud's disease if severe enough goes to necrosis of the finger tips and even more extensive gangrene when occlusion of the small vessels supervenes on vasoconstriction.

683 Acrocyanosis is a fairly common condition seen in young women. They have a characteristic blueish red coloration of the hands and feet sometimes with numbness and pain which is brought on by cold. The peripheral pulses are normal when the patient is warm.

684 Cervical outlet compression This may produce pressure on the subclavian artery or the brachial plexus. If on the artery the patient may experience ischaemic attacks in the hand. Radiography may show a cervical rib, which is illustrated here lying behind the artery.

681

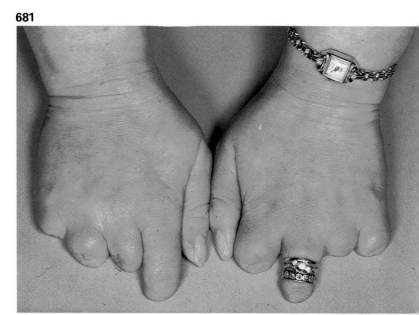

682

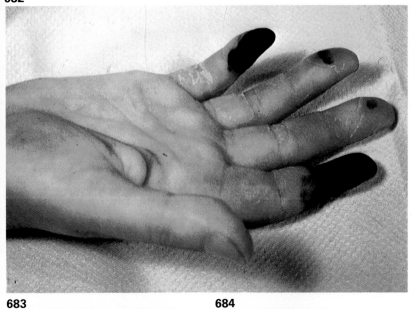

683

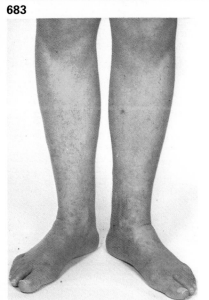

684

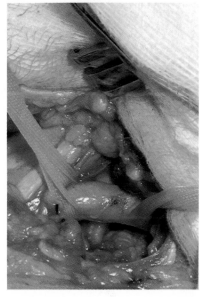

399

685 Cervical outlet compression This may be due to pressure from the scalaneus anterior or medius muscle and/or cervical rib, or the costo-clavicular syndrome where the space between the clavicle and first rib is narrow. The arteriogram illustrates the compression produced on abduction of the arm.

686 A torn brachial artery due to avulsion of the arm. The artery has sealed itself off.

687 Arteriovenous fistula This may be congenital as in this patient or acquired due to trauma. The illustration shows the swelling of an arterio-venous fistula in the medial half of the wrist and hand. It was soft, easily compressible, had a palpable thrill and machinery murmur and dilatation of the superficial veins.

688 Scleroderma This collagen disorder produces digital ischaemia due to thickening of the intima and perivascular fibrosis. The thickened skin is evident with coarseness of the hand and atrophy of the finger tips. Chronic painful ulcers may develop over the joints. The only features are stiffness of the joints, hyperhidrosis and the presence of Raynaud's phenomenon.

685

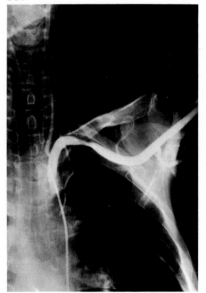

686

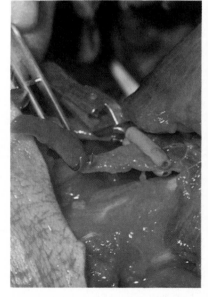

687

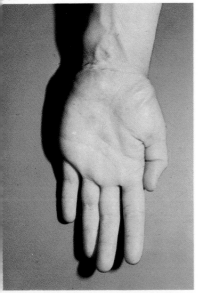

688

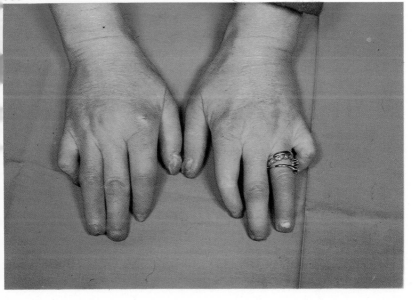

689 Trench feet was the name given to the severe ischaemia due to digital thrombosis brought on by exposure to cold and wet. This patient suffered in the trenches in the first world war.

689

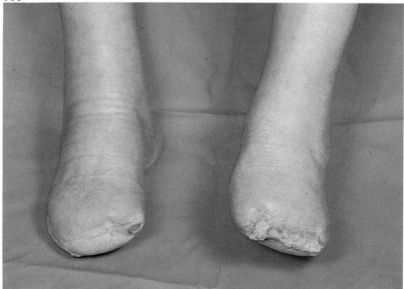

Disease of Veins and Lymphatics

690 Thrombophlebitis produces a reddened, tender, painful swelling of the veins. The affected veins are palpable and the redness may become diffuse.

691 Thrombophlebitis due to intravenous infusion. The patient complains of pain in the vein being infused especially if the fluid volume is increased. A red line passes upwards from the site of the needle or cannula.

690

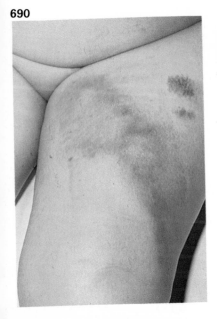

691

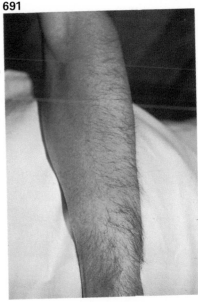

692 Varicose veins appear as tortuous dilated veins in the thigh and below the knee. A varix is visible at the upper end of the long saphenous vein. It disappears on elevation of the leg or direct pressure.

693 Saphena varix excised from the patient. This localised swelling in the vein is non-pulsatile, easily compressible and disappears on elevation of the limb and emptying of the veins.

694 Varicose dermatitis is seen in the lower leg especially on the medial side. Varicose veins are usually visible above the brownish red induration of the skin. The acute eczematous reaction shown here is the result of ointments or antibiotics applied to the area.

695 Varicose ulcers vary in depth and size. They are found in the ankle region and the associated veins are usually visible.

696 Chronic venous insufficiency can produce gross oedema and ulceration of the legs without visible superficial veins. The ulcer in this patient's right leg is circumferential producing a lymphatic stasis also and gross swelling of the foot.

692

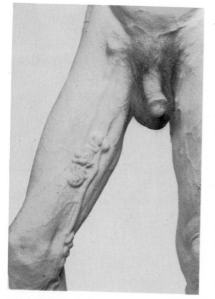

693

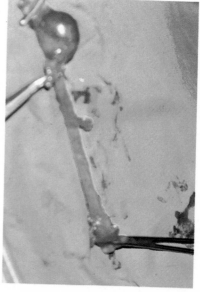

694

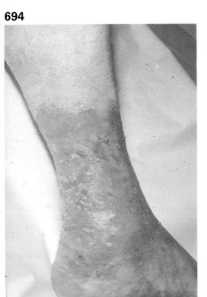

695

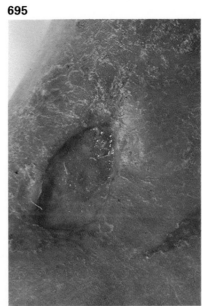

696

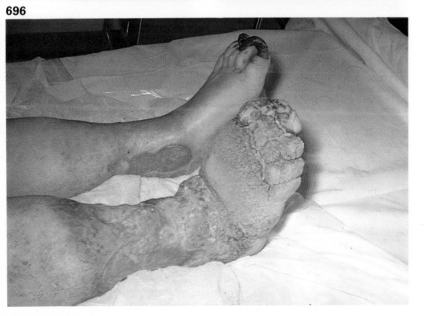

697 Deep vein thrombosis (phlegmasia alba dolens) The white leg describes the swelling and pitting oedema that follows iliofemoral vein thrombosis. Note the shiny skin in front of the left leg. The site of blockage may be confirmed by radiography.

698 Deep vein thrombosis (phlegmasia cerulea dolens) The painful blue leg is due to iliofemoral vein thrombosis and a degree of ischaemia. The leg is swollen, painful and the left foot was paler than the right. The pressure in the thigh in some cases is remarkable.

699 A deep vein thrombosis can affect the upper limb also as shown in the right arm in the patient (effort syndrome). The blockage of the right subclavian vein is shown on the x-ray. It was probably due to compression of the vein at the cervical outlet. The compression is made worse on elevation of the arm.

700 A superior vena caval thrombosis as shown by the distended neck veins and those on the chest wall. Confirmation came from venography. The young woman was on 'the pill'.

697

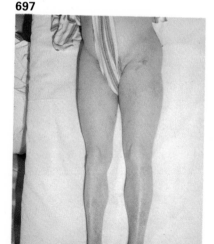

698

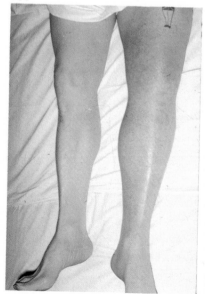

699

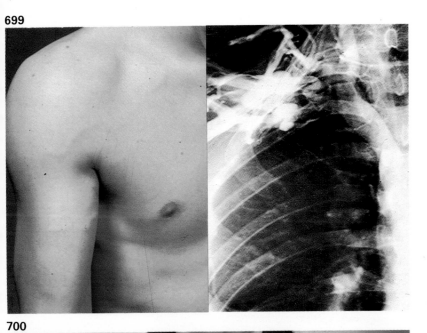

700

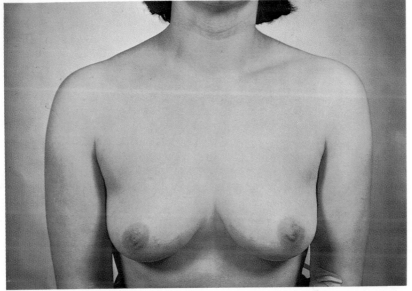

701 Lymphoedema (primary) is shown in the right leg. It had been present since childhood as a soft pitting oedema of foot and ankle gradually involving the whole leg.

702 Lymphoedema (secondary) The pitting oedema is shown as well as the biopsy site. The lymphatic glands were replaced by squamous carcinoma, the primary site of which was unknown.

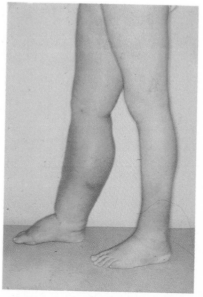

701

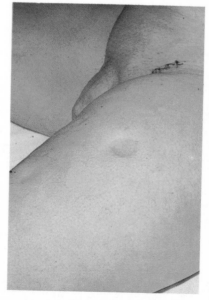

702

Disease of the Heart

Congenital heart disease

Developmental defects in the heart are present in about one per cent of newborn babies. Various factors are implicated: maternal rubella, chromosomal abnormalities and genetic defects, but it is difficult in the majority of cases to detect a cause.

Clinical diagnosis of the type of congenital cardiac lesion may be fairly easy but in the very young and those with complex lesions it can be very difficult. In these, cardiac catheterisation and cineangiocardiography will be necessary and indeed in most cases are valuable in indicating the severity of the condition and the need for operation.

There are many cardiac lesions, some of great complexity. The common ones only will be discussed.

As many of the severe lesions have a high initial mortality the incidence at birth differs from that seen in later childhood.

703 Ventricular septal defect is the commonest abnormality and may give rise to early heart failure in the first year of life. Otherwise poor growth and frequent respiratory infections occur associated with the increased pulmonary blood flow. A pan-systolic murmur is heard at the left sternal border. Cardiac catheterisation and angiography will establish the diagnosis, and indicate its serious nature. The cotton wool indicates the site of the vascular septal defect in the specimen.

703

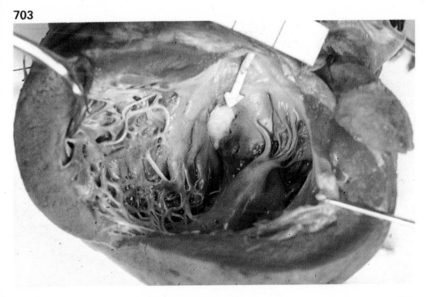

704 Atrial septal defect is of three types: Primum, secundum and complete atrio-ventricular canal. The common secundum defect may be asymptomatic. There is a right ventricular heave with splitting of the second sound and a pulmonary systolic murmur. The primum type often has an apical systolic murmur and left axis deviation on E.C.G. The A/V canal is the most serious with early heart failure, cardiomegaly, and a pansystolic murmur. The atrial septal defect is shown closed by sutures.

705 Pulmonary stenosis may be asymptomatic, or if severe produce right heart failure and cyanosis. There is a high pitched systolic ejection murmur in second left interspace and a marked right ventricular heave. The ballooning of the pulmonary valve area is visible on angiography indicating valvular obstruction.

706 Patent ductus arteriosus may be detected by the auscultation of a continuous murmur in second left interspace and a loud second heart sound. If large the infant may be poorly developed with recurrent chest infections. In these the machinery murmur may be replaced by a systolic murmur in the pulmonary area.

707 Aortic stenosis may be asymptomatic or if severe produce angina and syncope or heart failure. There is a prominent left ventricular impulse and a narrow pulse pressure. A thrill can be felt along the left sternal border and a harsh systolic murmur with a systolic ejection click is heard there. Angiocardiography will distinguish the four types: stenotic valve, supravalvular and subvalular stenosis and hypertrophied subaortic muscle. The angiogram shows valvular stenosis, ballooning and post-stenotic dilatation.

704

705

706

707

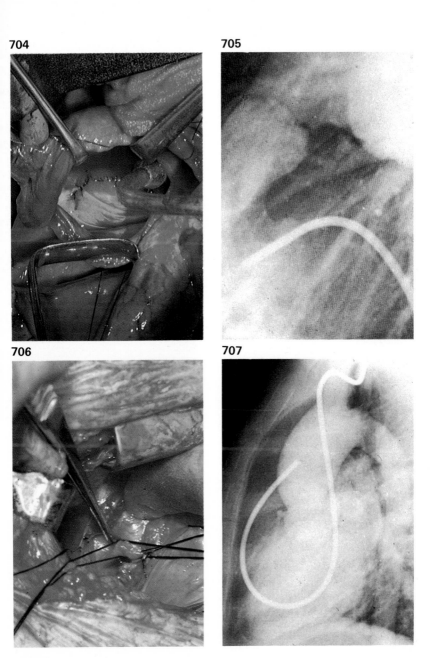

411

708 Coarctation of the aorta may be detected at birth by noting the absence of or markedly diminished, femoral pulses. If mild there may be no symptoms; if severe, cardiac failure may develop. The differences in the limb pressures can be measured and a harsh systolic murmur is heard in the back.

709 Coarctation of aorta This is a section of the aorta removed showing the very tiny eccentric opening. Small wonder the peripheral pulses are absent or very diminished.

710 Tetralogy of Fallot consists of a large ventricular septal defect, pulmonary stenosis, an over-riding aorta and hypertrophy of the right ventricle. The patient is cyanotic and has marked clubbing of the fingers. There is a prominent right ventricular impulse and an ejection murmur in the third left intercostal space.

708

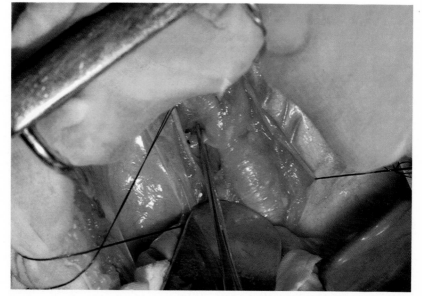

709

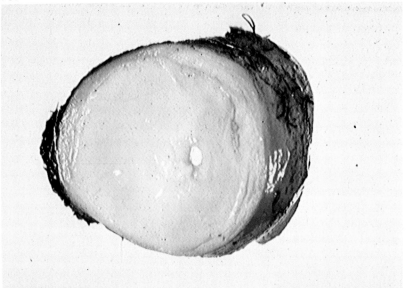

710

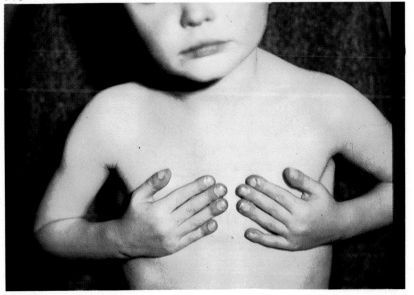

413

711 Tetralogy of Fallot The squatting position shown here brings relief to the child who may suffer from attacks of increased cyanosis and syncope.

712 Transposition of the great vessels is another type of cyanotic heart disease. Heart failure in infancy is common. Auscultation is not helpful as the murmur can vary. The child is often thought to have the tetralogy of Fallot and the final diagnosis is established by cardioangiography which shows the aorta arising from the anterior ventricle.

711

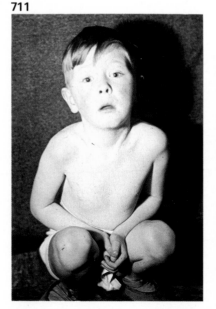

712

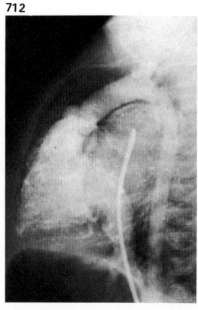

Acquired heart disease

713 Mitral stenosis is the most common heart lesion and is secondary to rheumatic fever. Due to the narrowed valve there is increasing back pressure on the lungs with dyspnoea on effort, orthopnoea and paroxysmal nocturnal dyspnoea. The first apical heart sound is loud with opening snap and a crescendo diastolic rumble. X-ray may show prominent pulmonary vessels with perhaps pulmonary congestion and an enlarged left atrium. The heart is shown cut transversely, the narrow mitral valve lower left of the specimen.

714 Mitral stenosis A close up view of the mitral valve to show the very narrow orifice of less than 1 cm and the fusion of the cusps.

713

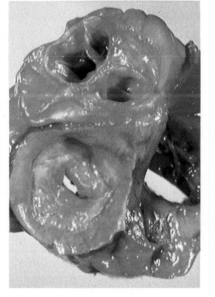

714

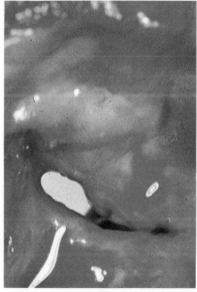

715 Mitral regurgitation is due to incompetence of the valve which is seen here on close-up to be thoroughly disorganised. Calcification is seen on the anterolateral border of the opening. Clinically this produces marked pulmonary congestion with severe dyspnoea. A loud systolic murmur is heard at the apex radiating into the axilla. Radiography may show a giant sized left atrium and left ventricular dilatation.

716 Mitral regurgitation This valve was removed at operation and a prosthesis inserted. The margins of the opening are irregular. The anterior cusp (lower one) was thickened and shortened and the posterior one very much fibrosed.

717 Aortic stenosis is shown in the centre of the specimen with the pulmonary valve anteriorly and the mitral and tricuspid behind. Clinically the patient may suffer from syncopal attacks or angina during exercise. A systolic ejection type murmur is heard in the second right interspace transmitted up into the neck. Radiography may show calcification of the valve and an enlarged left ventricle.

715

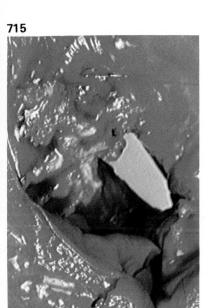

716

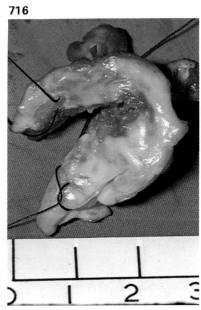

717

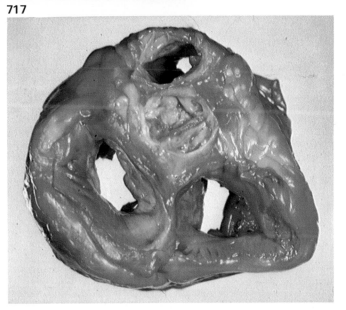

417

718 Aortic regurgitation The gross distortion of the aortic valve is apparent. This may at first be tolerated without much trouble but decompensation can occur quickly with rapidly increasing left heart failure and pulmonary congestion and oedema. There will be a marked left ventricular heave and a collapsing pulse. The apex is displaced into the axilla and a diminuendo blowing diastolic murmur is heard in second right interspace.

719 Coronary artery disease produces narrowing of the coronary arteries with cardiac ischaemia characterised by an oppressive pain across the front of the chest on exercise or stress. The pain is relieved by rest or nitroglycerine – angina pectoris. E.C.G. may show changes especially after mild exercise.

720 Ventricular aneurysm follows on a large myocardial infarct which scars up instead of rupturing. The scar stretches to produce the aneurysm which is recognised on straight x-ray as a bulge on the left ventricular border. E.C.G. changes are fairly typical and cineangiography will establish the diagnosis.

718

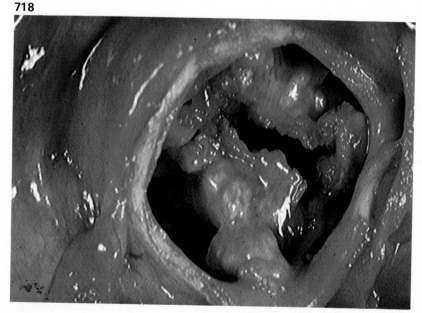

719

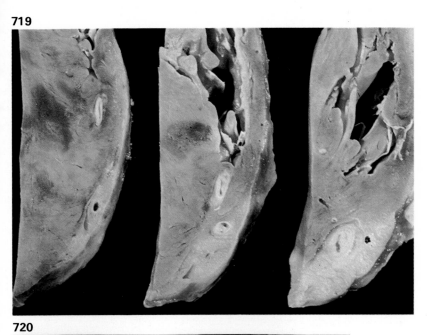

720

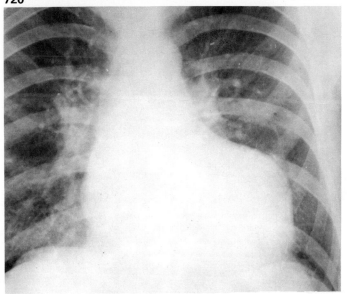

721 Dissecting aneurysm of aorta This presents often as a sudden severe tearing pain in the chest with radiation into the back and down into the abdomen. Hypertension or the signs of Marfan's syndrome may be present. Radiography shows the broadened aortic arch with pleural effusion. Angiography may help to establish the diagnosis.

722 Thoracic aortic aneurysms are usually fusiform dilatations of the lumen but may be saccular especially in the syphilitic. Enlargement causes pressure effects on the sternum and vertebra with pain and on the recurrent laryngeal nerve with hoarseness. X-ray shows an enlarged mediastinum.

723 Angiography of the same aneurysm shows the dilatation of the aorta. The erosion of the vertebral bodies is obvious.

724 Constrictive pericarditis The thickened adherent pericardium is demonstrated here being removed at operation. It produces a reduced cardiac output with distension of the jugular veins and a raised right atrial pressure. Calcification may be visible on x-ray.

721

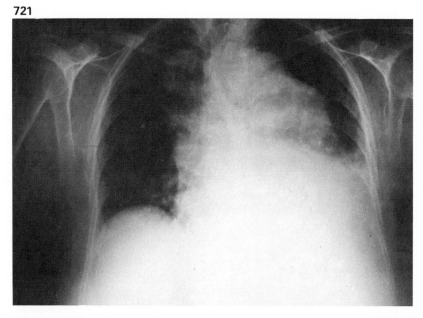

722

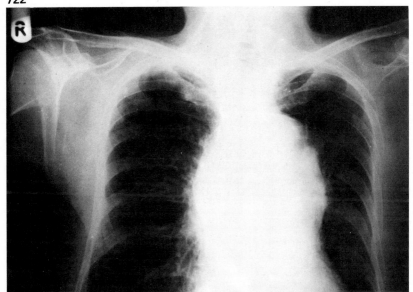

723

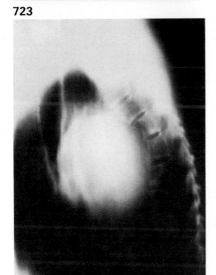

724

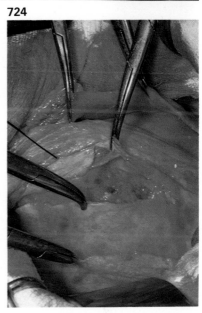

Cardiac tumours

These are fortunately rare but can occur at any age. Benign tumours account for 75% of all these tumours, of them the commonest is the myxoma.

725 Cardiac myxoma The clinical features are variable. The tumour in this patient was producing ball-valve obstruction of the mitral valve with signs suggestive of mitral stenosis. The diagnosis was established at operation when a hard mass was felt in the left atrium. A fragmenting tumour may cause peripheral arterial embolisation.

725

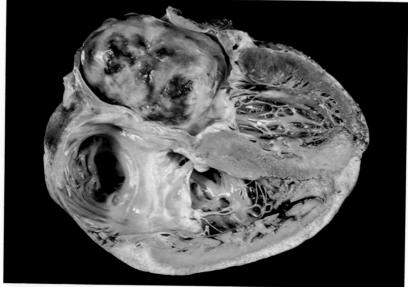

Chest Trauma

726 Subcutaneous emphysema is the result of air infiltrating the subcutaneous tissues and produces this typical picture of a bloated individual. Crepitus is felt on pressure. It may follow trauma to the lungs or leakage of air along a drainage tube.

727 Traumatic asphyxia is the rupture of small vessels due to sudden massive compression of the chest. Subconjunctival haemorrhages seen here may be associated with haemorrhages of the skin.

726

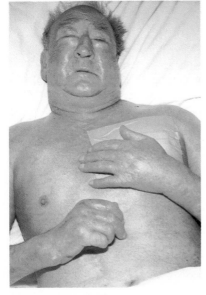

727

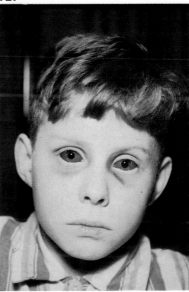

728 Fracture of the ribs may follow a direct blow or a crush injury. Several ribs are broken on the right side and a pleural effusion is present. They cause pain on movement or coughing and if multiple, instability of the chest wall. The fragments may injure blood vessels or lung producing a haemothorax or pneumothorax.

729 Pneumothorax There is almost total collapse of the left lung and the left chest is full of air. This is a spontaneous one not due to trauma. The chest on that side is hyper-resonant and breath sounds are absent. An intercostal drain allowed escape of air and reflation of the lung.

730 Haemothorax bleeding into the pleural cavity may or may not be associated with accumulation of air. It follows trauma, operation, neoplasm and rupture of vessels. Pain and shock may be present. Aspiration by a needle will settle the diagnosis.

728

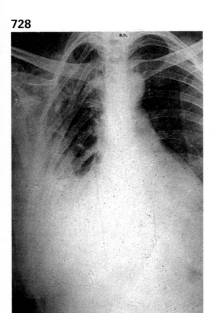

729

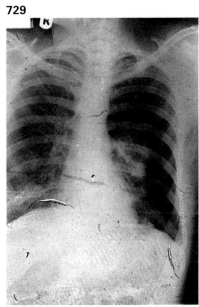

730

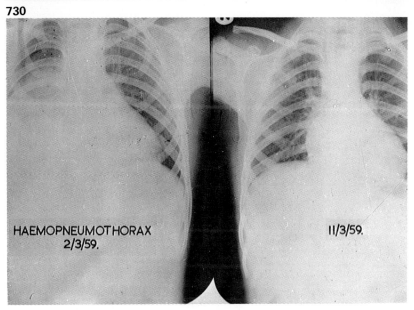

HAEMOPNEUMOTHORAX
2/3/59.

11/3/59.

425

731 A stab wound of chest is unfortunately a common emergency. The knife shown here has not penetrated the heart and has not produced a pneumothorax or effusion. Diagnosis is more difficult if the instrument is removed and one is left with a wound in the chest wall. Exploration depends on further progress of the patient in these cases.

732 A foreign body in a bronchus as shown in the right side may be known by the history or suspected when there is a sudden onset of pain, coughing, cyanosis. Teeth may be a cause following head injuries. A lateral x-ray of chest should always be done as the foreign body may be hidden by the sternum or vertebrae.

733 Fat embolism may follow injury especially to the long bones. This patient collapsed after operative reduction of a fracture of tibia and fibula. Tiny petechiae were noted in the neck and lower eyelid.

734 Tiny petechiae in lower eyelid supported diagnosis of fat embolism.

735 Rupture of diaphragm may result from compression of chest and abdomen. The intestine is apparent above the normal level of the diaphragm.

731

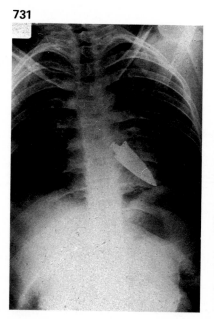

732

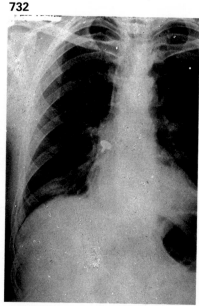

733

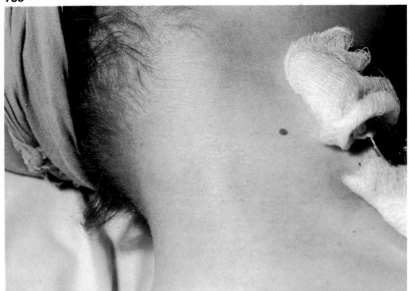

734

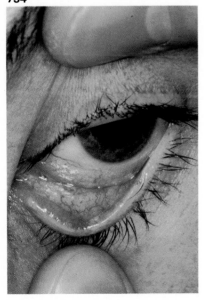

735

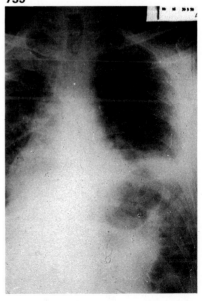

Post-operative pulmonary complications

These vary from an exacerbation of a previous bronchitis to fatal pulmonary embolism. Some of the lesions may be combined.

736 Aspiration pneumonia occurred in the patient who had an intestinal obstruction and inhaled some vomitus. He became breathless and cyanosed. Coarse crepitations were heard on ausculation and diminished air entry. On x-ray patchy areas are seen in the right lung.

737 Extreme aspiration damage to the lungs and a hugely distended stomach are shown. The patient had just delivered a child and inhaled vomit thereafter. She collapsed, became breathless and cyanosed. The reaction to the inhalation of acid gastric juice is sometimes termed Mendelson's syndrome.

736

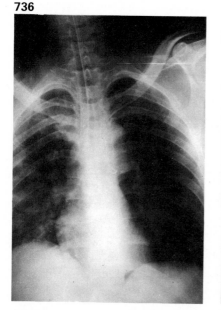

737

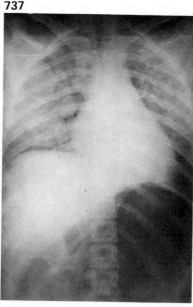

738 Atelectasis may vary from minor areas of collapse of the lung to more massive collapse. Following operation the patient is not as well as expected. There may be a slight pyrexia, tachycardia dyspnoea and a hint of cyanosis around the lips. Breath sounds are diminished on the affected side. In this case radiography demonstrated the degree of atelectasis affecting the right upper and middle lobe. Improvement was complete within two weeks.

738

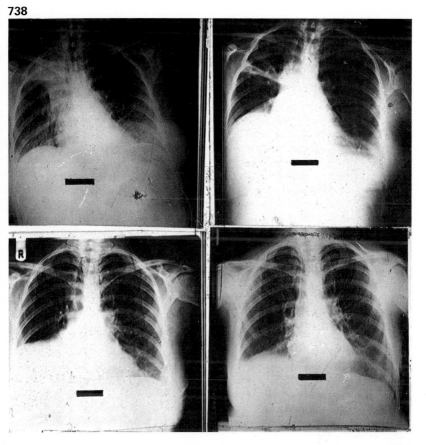

739 Lung abscess may follow pneumonia or atelectasis. There is a marked pyrexia, tachycardia and dyspnoea. The patient looks ill and on x-ray an area of consolidation is seen with a fluid level.

740 Empyema is the presence of pus in the pleural cavity and may follow a lung abscess or be due to infection of a pleural effusion or haemothorax. Pyrexia, tachycardia, dyspnoea and a limited air entry may suggest the diagnosis. The lateral x-ray shows a fluid level.

741 Empyema This is usually intrapleural, especially following operations such as oesophagectomy. In this patient who had a ligature of a patent ductus arteriosus, the empyema developed in the extrapleural space probably as a result of an infected blood clot in the region of the thoracotomy.

742 Pulmonary oedema is well known in cardiac failure but may occur also in the management of difficult chest lesions perhaps on the respirator. Excess of I.V. fluids, infection of the lung, and cardiac failure play their part. The patient is distressed, dyspnoeic, may pour out fluid from the mouth or endotracheal tube, and has the characteristic picture shown on x-ray.

739

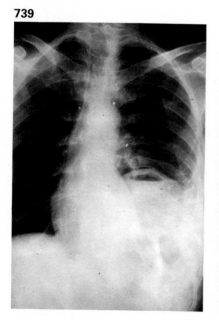

740

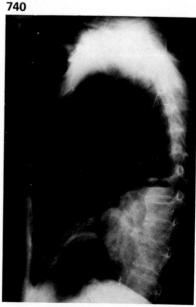

741

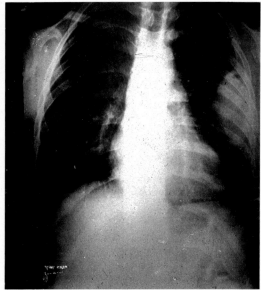

742

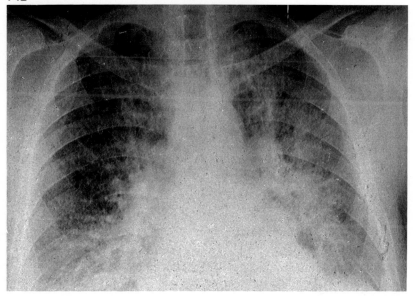

743 Pulmonary embolism may occur in all grades of severity from the subclinical to that resulting in rapid death. A cough with a bloody spit and pain may be present or sudden collapse with constrictive feeling in the chest and severe dyspnoea. X-ray may show diminished vascularity of a segment of lung.

744 Pulmonary embolism Angiography may show a complete block in a pulmonary artery as seen here in the left side. E.C.G. is helpful.

745 Pulmonary embolectomy was carried out in a woman seven days post-parturition. This was done by Trendelenburg method; i.e. clamping the vena cavae, incising the pulmonary trunk, and removal of these clots.

743

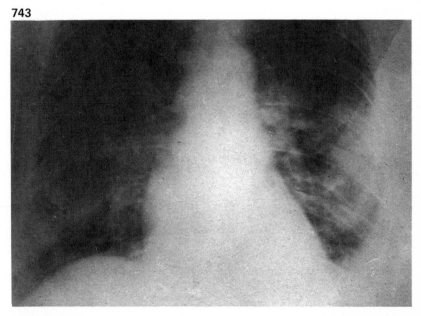

744

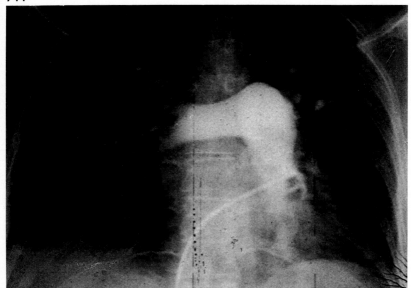

745

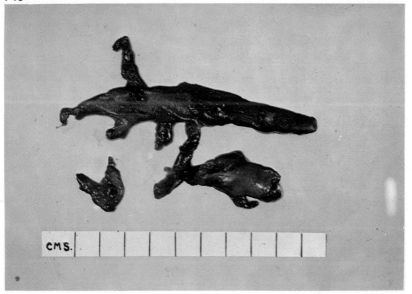

CMS.

Head Injuries

Haemorrhages

746 Extradural haematoma is due to injury to the anterior or posterior branches of the middle meningeal artery or to rupture of the venous sinuses. The blow may be minor with a short period of unconsciousness, perhaps not noticed, followed perhaps by lucid interval then unconsciousness and neurological changes. The blood clots are usually in the temporal area.

747 Subdural haematoma The symptoms depend on the magnitude of the bleeding from the veins so that the haematoma may be acute, subacute or chronic. The acute form develops within hours of the injury and is similar to the extradural type except there is no fracture of the skull. The subacute form occurs within days and the chronic form is weeks to months. The clot exposed at operation was deep to the dura.

748 Intracerebral haemorrhage may be subcortical and small or major haemorrhage from a large vessel, as here. There is no clear-cut picture. The signs and symptoms are due to an expanding lesion.

746

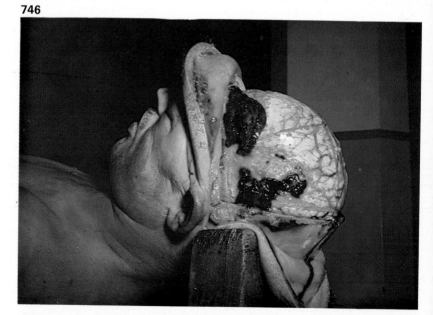

747

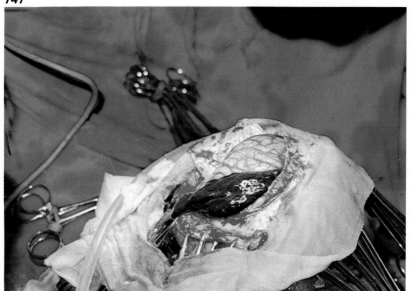

748

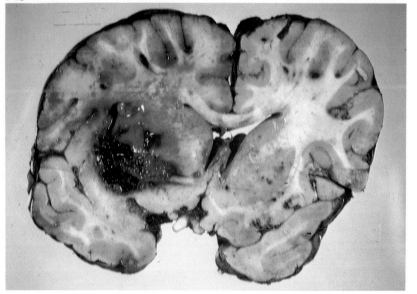

Fractures of skull

749 Fracture of vault may be due to compression or direct or tangential blows from large or small objects. These produce different types of fractures. Apart from compound injuries the next important fracture is the one overlying the branch of the middle meningeal vessels as shown in **746**. An extradural haemorrhage was the result.

750 Fracture of anterior fossa may produce rhinorrhoea, or if it extends into the orbit, a typical discoloration is seen round the eyes. It usually appears some hours after injury and is not associated with damage to the periorbital skin as would be seen in a typical 'black eye'.

751 Fracture of anterior fossa with subconjunctival haemorrhage. Typically the extent of the backward spread of the haemorrhage cannot be seen. In a 'black eye' or other cause of haemorrhage the posterior limit is usually visible.

752 Fracture of posterior and middle fossae were due in this case to a motor car accident. Blood and C.S.F. were discharged from the ear and a boggy swelling below the occiput suggested presence of a posterior fossa fracture.

749

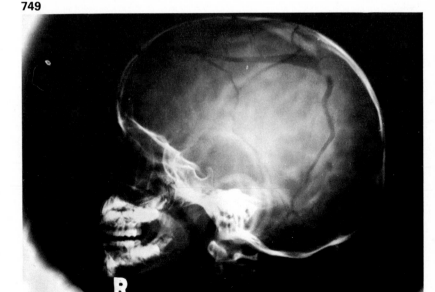

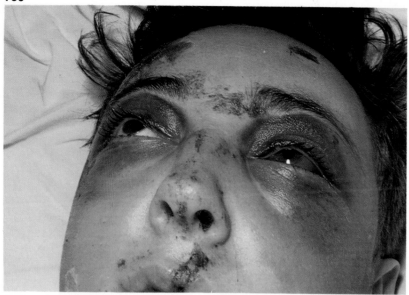

750

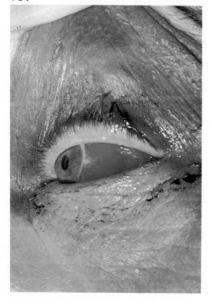

751

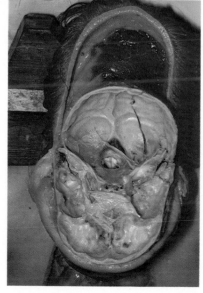

752

Fractures of face

753 Fracture of nose This common injury is detected by pain, swelling and tenderness over the root of the nose. A finger run over the bridge of the nose may detect a sharp break. The index fingers on either side may detect the deformity in the general swelling and also mobility of the bones and crepitus. Deviation of the nose or injury to the spetum require early manipulation.

754 Fracture of zygoma This may be hidden in the general swelling and bruising of the soft tissues and may only be detected by x-ray. Flattening of the malar bone on one side of the face and if present irregularity or mobility of the bones will be diagnostic.

755 Fracture of maxilla and left zygoma This followed a beating. The bruising of the left side of the face is evident with bleeding from the nose and bilateral black eyes. Fracture confirmed by x-ray.

756 Bilateral maxillary fractures ('dishface') This produces a rather typical 'frog face' appearance when the centre portion of the face is pushed back. This type of injury may be seen when the face hits the windscreen of a car.

753

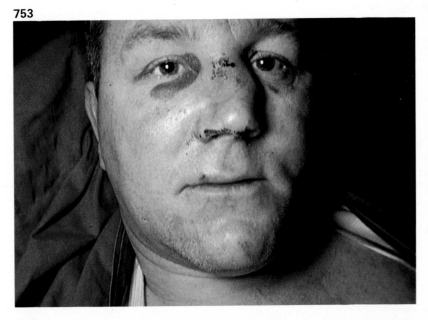

754

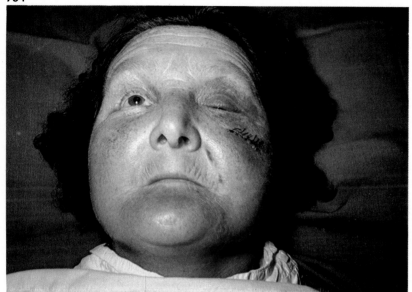

755

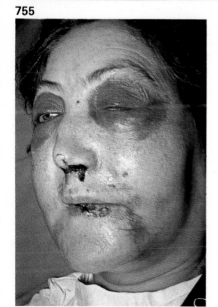

756

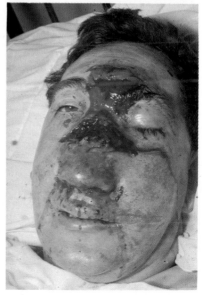

757 Fracture of mandible due to direct trauma. The patient was struck on the face with a sharp piece of metal which produced a compound injury of his maxilla. The mandible appeared uneven on palpation. A fracture was confirmed by x-ray.

757

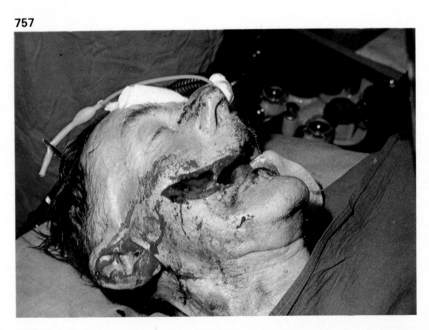

Index

(References printed in italic type are to page numbers and those in **bold** are to picture and caption numbers.)